PERFECT DRINKING
and its
ENEMIES

PERFECT

DRINKING

and its

ENEMIES

Kari Poikolainen

A wise man proportions his belief to the evidence.

David Hume

Second edition

Revised and updated

© Kari Poikolainen 2013 and 2020

All rights reserved. No part of this publication may be reproduced, stored in retrieval system, or transmitted, in any form or by any means, without the prior permission in writing of Kari Poikolainen, or as expressly permitted by law, by license or under terms agreed with the appropriate reprographics rights organization. Inquiries concerning reproduction outside the scope of the above should be sent to poikolainen47@gmail.com.

First edition Mill City Press 2014

Second edition, updated and revised 2020.

ISBN: 9798635577844

Disclaimer

This book is intended as a reference volume only, not a medical manual. The information given here is designed to help you make informed decisions regarding your health. It is not intended as a substitute for any treatment that may have been prescribed by your doctor. If you suspect that you have a medical problem, I urge you to seek competent medical help.

Mention of specific companies, individuals, organizations, or authorities does not necessarily imply that they endorse this book, its author, or the publisher. Internet addresses and links provided in this book were accurate at the time when accessed.

CONTENTS

INTRODUCTION - THE VIRTUE AND ITS ENEMIES........5

 The second edition..8

 Acknowledgments..9

 List of tables..9

 List of figures..9

 List of abbreviations..10

I..13

ENJOY AND PROMOTE YOUR HEALTH..........................13

 2 *Are alcoholic beverages good for health? - Yes, when enjoyed in moderation*..16

  The lower the mortality, the longer the life-span............16

  Drinking rhythm and health..26

 3 *What is the risk level of alcohol intake? - More indulgent than you have been told*..32

  Make your own rules..41

  Moral implications of risk..42

 4 *The good effects of moderation are real - despite what the anti-alcohol academics say*..45

  Randomized trials..50

  Genetic studies..54

  Animal experiments..57

  Blood pressure..57

II..59

UNDER THE INFLUENCE - BLOOD ALCOHOL AND ACUTE EFFECTS..59

5 *The rise and fall of blood alcohol*..................................61

6 *The acute effects - Feeling good, feeling bad*..................68

The good effects...70

7 Not only a poison...72

III..75

THE DRINKS – HEALTH AND GOOD TASTE..................75

8 *Water - The essence of life*................................77

The taste of good water..................................78

9 *Wine, beer and liquor - The milk of adults*......................80

10 *Coffee, tea and energy drinks - The soft stimulants*.......83

11 *What is good taste*..86

From stimuli to perception................................86

Tasting performance......................................88

Dimensions of taste..90

12 *Should teenagers be allowed to taste alcoholic beverages*
- Consider carefully..93

IV...97

PROTECT YOURSELF...97

13 *Avoid AUDIT and brief advice in health care*..............100

Brief advice wastes resources and may be hazardous to
health...103

How should I respond?...106

14 *Count and record your own alcohol intake*..................108

V..111

RISKS, HIGH AND LOW.......................................111

15 *The many causes of liver cirrhosis*..............................114

16 *Some cancers are alcohol-related*............................118

Breast cancer...120

17 Gout - The revenge of affluence..................122

18 Aggression and violence-The devil within.................125

Aggressive behavior depends on culture.................126

19 Traffic accidents - Drinkers drive better.................128

20 Harms to the unborn - Is there a safe drinking level and what are the causes of fetal alcohol syndrome.................131

Facial and other anomalies.................132

Growth deficit.................133

Central nervous system abnormalities.................133

Risk level.................134

Causes of fetal alcohol syndrome and related diagnoses 135

Panic, politics and warning labels.................136

VI...139

ALCOHOLISM - THE RAGE TO ENJOY.................139

21 The disease concept.................143

Disease as a social construction.................146

22 Biomedical views on the cause of addiction.................149

The role of genes is exaggerated.................149

The false step of the animal experiment.................151

The tenets of the present biomedical models have been proven wrong.................152

23 From general principles to risk factors.................155

Voluntary choices.................157

Willpower.................160

Risk factors.................161

The bad habit loop..164

"Natural" and self-help recovery..................................167

24 The unknown value of professional treatment...............169

VII...173

WHAT AILS THE DOMINANT ALCOHOL POLICY
THEORIES..173

25 The size of the problem - Inflated figures sell best.......175

The problem of alcohol-specific diseases.....................176

Cost of harm estimates – good for indoctrination........178

The underlying logic of cost-of-alcohol harm studies..179

26 Errors in the dominant theory....................................181

The skewed distribution...184

Heavy drinkers and harm...185

Price and alcohol consumption...................................189

A fresh look at alcohol policy.....................................196

REFERENCES...199

INTRODUCTION - THE VIRTUE AND ITS ENEMIES

This book is about health, enjoyment and drinking, from water to hard liquor. It aims to inform you so that you can decide how drinking is likely to be best for you. It tells what you need to know about the facts, common errors and frequent misunderstandings. The latter two abound. And please, consider the evidence and draw your own conclusions.

There are four enemies of perfect drinking: abstinence, alcoholism, inadequate information and myopic alcohol policies. For most of us, moderate drinking is better than abstinence. Moderate amounts can be higher than the guidelines say. However, exceeding these guidelines may result in the false label of alcoholism if you do not protect yourself. Part IV deals with protecting yourself and Part VI with what alcoholism really is. Some people have good moral or health reasons for abstinence. Let us respect them and feel compassion for alcoholics but follow the path of moderation.

Much of the available information on alcohol is hard to grasp and a great deal of it biased. More often than not, the harmful effects of alcoholic beverages are exaggerated and the benefits disparaged or denied. Protect yourself from misleading claims, often presented with expert authority and with the best possible intentions. Well-meant advice can undermine your health.

6

A major enemy resides in the anti-alcohol movement. It is an informally organized lobby active in influencing politicians, international organizations, health professions and the public. This is fine when the argumentation is honest and based on facts. However, there is also foul play around.

The dark side favors three tools: manipulation of evidence, dogma construction and witch-hunting. Scientific evidence is manipulated to strengthen the views of the movement and then presented as the final truth. Some manipulation can be revealed by the careful reading of research papers and other publications. From the beginning of my research career I was advised to read studies thoroughly and assess them critically. This has allowed me to detect some of the errors found in published studies. This, however, only scratches the surface. I suspect that more remain hidden. Research findings can be tampered with, fabricated or left unpublished.[1]

Those who do not accept the current dogmas are accused of being underlings of the alcohol trade. Suspicions are aroused if the scientist has any relations with the trade. In many cases

---

[1]

Fraud in science is likely to be an important source of erroneous results, although it is difficult to prove. According to 21 surveys, 2 % of responding scientists admit falsifying or fabricating data, but 28 % claimed to know of colleagues who engaged in questionable research practices (Unreliable research, The Economist, October 19 - 25, 2013:21-24).

7

the transgression is only to receive a research grant from an independent scientific foundation funded to some extent by the business.

Labeling scientists who do not accept the dogma as trade sidekicks aims to discredit troublesome findings. Witch-hunting is the easy way, since no scientific argumentation is needed. The movement tries to prevent funding and publication of studies they disagree with. Some scientific journals are under the control of the anti-alcohol lobby. Typically, these journals were originally run by temperance organizations. The anti-alcohol movement is a continuation of the militant temperance movement and is fed by the distortions in lobbying by the alcohol trade. It champions misleading alcohol policies.

I retired from the post of Research Director at the Finnish Foundation for Alcohol Studies to write this book because I suspected that some generally accepted views were false or rested on weak ground. Review of the literature has shown that this is indeed the case.

Only a small part of the literature I've read is mentioned in the references, those that are most recent, most pivotal or most illustrative in my opinion. Pivotal studies are often the unique of their kind. They change the way we see things and should be praised because of this.

A search for truth motivates this book. I believe that the final truth about the issues dealt with here is unattainable but that a down-to-earth summary can be reached based on the current findings. This includes estimating the degree of uncertainty of our knowledge today. I hope that this book will benefit those enjoying and interested in drinking. I also hope that it will inspire others to improve on the present work. I have received no funding or other support for this book from any enterprise producing, distributing, selling or advertising alcoholic beverages or drugs, neither from the alcoholism treatment industry nor from any other source.

The second edition

The seven parts can be read as independent essays. The chapter structure remains the same. Most relevant recent research has been reviewed as well as new insights from older work. Larger changes pertain to the health effects and alcohol policy.

My aim is to provide facts to the interested reader who seeks to form her or his independent opinion on the issues at hand. Therefore, I felt it necessary to give a fair amount of background information as well as explain concepts and methods that are familiar to scientists but not the general reader.

I have tried to maintain a balanced view. It is for the reader to judge how far I have succeeded. In my view, the arguments put forward in the first edition have generally received greater support while others called for further honing. When revising the book, I have been impressed by how ancient Stoic philosophy has antedated modern views of self-control

9

and peace of mind.

I wish to dedicate this edition to the memory of Kettil Bruun (1924 ~ 1985). He was my mentor and a man with honesty and dignity, unafraid to change his opinion when justified by new facts.

Kari Poikolainen

Acknowledgments

I thank statistical consultant John Duffy for his comments, and Jon Beasley for editing the language. The views expressed herein are solely those of the author. Any errors rest upon my shoulders alone.

List of tables

Table 1. Alcohol intake and relative risk of death according to a meta-analysis

Table 2. Number of 10 g drinks, number of drinking days and the relative risk of coronary heart disease (lifelong abstainers = 1).

Table 3. AUDIT-C questions and scoring

Table 4. Approximate pH values for some drinks

List of figures

Figure 1. Alcohol and mortality - a theoretical model

Figure 2. Alcohol and relative risk: regular 7/7 (black curve) and irregular 3/7 (gray curve) days a week rhythm

Figure 3. Blood alcohol curve variation after equal dose of alcohol as liquor, portwine, table wine or beer

Figure 4. Blood alcohol curve variation after equal dose of alcohol as table wine or beer with or without food

List of abbreviations

ADH	Alcohol dehydrogenase
ALT	Alanine transaminase
ALDH	Acetaldehyde dehydrogenase
AST	Aspartate transaminase
BAC	Blood alcohol concentration
CHD	Coronary heart disease
CI	Confidence interval
DALY	Disability-adjusted life year
DSM	Diagnostic and Statistical Manual of Mental Disorders
g	gram
GGT	Gamma-glutamyltransferase
HDL	High-density lipoprotein (cholesterol)
ICD	International Classification of Diseases, Injuries and Causes of Death
kcal	kilocalorie

11

LDL	Low-density lipoprotein (cholesterol)
RR	Relative risk, risk ratio
WHO	World Health Organization

12

I

ENJOY AND PROMOTE YOUR HEALTH

14

In the 20th century, there were two very-well known men who both were avid painters and verbally talented. One was a great drinker and smoker, the other a vegetarian, non-smoker and abstainer. Who would you think had the longer life-span? The first lived for 90 years, the second shot himself at the age of 56 years. If you do not accept this comparison, let us take an American teetotaler and millionaire who lived for 97 years. Vivid examples of such famous people or our relatives often color our perceptions of the relation between habits and life-span, even if these comparisons are haphazard and extraordinary. The best available evidence comes from follow-up studies on large population groups. Let us review these more illuminating studies. But before that, have you found the names of the famous men? They are Sir Winston Churchill (Time magazine man of the half-century 1949), Adolf Hitler (Time magazine man of the year in 1938) and John D. Rockefeller (the man vilified by the press who could have bought Time magazine but instead gave huge sums to charity and education).

Alcohol has both good and bad effects on health. You might achieve either, depending on the choices you make. But this is not easy. There is an abundance of information, much of it difficult to comprehend without the basics of epidemiologic research. Let us examine these basics, review the most relevant studies and sum up.

First, the major studies and how they came about are described. A general model is then sketched, focusing on two

15

features of alcohol intake - quantity and rhythm. Part II tells how the speed of drinking affects behavior. The special features of beer, wine, liquor, water, coffee and tea are presented in Part III. As to health, it is best to limit ourselves mainly to the comprehensive attributes - life-span, self-reported health and the incidence of any disease or other ill-health. This is followed by a review of major diseases where alcohol intake can be beneficial. The major detriments will be presented in Part V.

To help you decide if there really are beneficial effects, we'll see how the research findings were brought about and discuss possible biases critically. We will end up by giving best estimates of risk levels. You'll be surprised.

2 Are alcoholic beverages good for health? - Yes, when enjoyed in moderation

Three aspects of alcohol intake - amount, rhythm and speed - determine whether the outcome is beneficial or harmful.

The Scottish writer James Hogg (1770 ~ 1835) suggested that if you could find the exact amount that ought to be drunk every day and put this wisdom into practice, you might live forever, thus making physicians and graveyards unfashionable. Alas, drinking is not able to take us this far, but it can help us to improve our health and lengthen our life-span. Both higher intake and abstinence promise shorter life and more disease. The present evidence points in that direction. But how good is it? Should you believe it? Let us review it to help you make up your mind.

The lower the mortality, the longer the life-span

How do we find information about alcohol and life-span? We could observe people and their drinking until they die. However, that would take too long, so that a more practical method is needed. And we have it, since the reverse of life-span is mortality. They are a bit like the two sides of the same coin. Suppose that you have 100 one-cent coins in your wallet and you will take every year one out to buy something.

17

Leaving the wallet is like a death for a coin. Mortality is the ratio of number of coins leaving the wallet to the number of coins remaining there in any given year. Because one coin leaves the wallet every year and the number of coins remaining there decreases the mortality rate increases every year. The average "life-span" in this population of coins in the wallet is approximately 50 years. This is just to give a rough idea about the relation between mortality and life-span. In human populations the relation is more complex but we do not have to go into the mathematics to understand the principle. However, a cautionary note must be presented.

Mortality data can be applied to calculate life-spans for different ages. For newborns it is called life expectancy at birth. The calculations are commonly based on current life tables, which describe the survival pattern of a hypothetical group of individuals (usually 100,000 persons) subject to death rates (specific for age, sex and possibly other factors) currently observed in a particular community within a particular time period. The calculations imply that no change in mortality takes place in future. Life span calculations are related to mortality but not in a straightforward way.[2]

---

[2] In a life-table population with a positive age-specific force of mortality at all ages, the expectation of life at age x is the average of the reciprocal of the survival-specific force of mortality at ages after x, weighted by life-table deaths at each age after x. Equivalently, the expectation of life when the surviving fraction in the life table is s is the average of the

18

Everybody is mortal, but mortality is not 100 percent because we all do not die at the same point in time. Mortality is the number of deaths in a population divided by the time persons in the same population have spent alive. Take one year and a population of 100,000 persons. If 600 persons die during this year, the person-years spent alive in this population is 99,400 (those who survive) plus 300 (assuming that the deaths are evenly spread over the year, leaving an average of 0.5 year spent alive for the deceased). The mortality rate in this population and in this year is then 600 per 99,700 person-years, that is 601.8 per 100,000 person-years. And the average life-span in this population is 0.997 years in this particular year. In the same vein we can calculate rates for the onset of disease. This is called the incidence of disease. Mortality is the incidence of death. These are the tools we need to describe the risks of death and disease. It took a long time before these tools were first used to study the effects of alcohol.

The temperance movement was born some two hundred years ago. It soon assumed a radical form and condemned all kinds of alcohol use. Any drinking was thought to cause misery and premature death. Down with the demon drink, a paradise

---

reciprocal of the survival-specific force of mortality over surviving proportions less than s, weighted by life-table deaths at surviving proportions less than s. See Cohen JE. Life expectancy is the death-weighted average of the reciprocal of the survival-specific force of mortality. *Demographic Research* 2010;22:115-128.

19

waits us! The movement became international and brought about prohibitions in many countries. During the Prohibition in the USA, a pivotal study refuted the claim on premature death. Raymond Pearl (1879 ~ 1940) studied white and blue-collar workers in Baltimore and found that moderate drinkers had lower mortality than abstainers or heavy drinkers (Pearl 1926). Among men aged 30 years, the percentage of deaths before the age of 60 years was as follows (my calculations based on the original data):

- abstainers   32%
- occasional moderate drinkers   36%
- steady moderate drinkers   29%
- occasional heavy drinkers   32%
- steady heavy drinkers   57%

The respective percentages for women were

- abstainers   30%
- occasional moderate drinkers   24%
- steady moderate drinkers   28%
- heavy drinkers   65%

Pearl's study had many strengths. The study population was large, 3,084 men and 2,164 women. To be classified as a moderate drinker, one should not become intoxicated and drink not more than three beers daily. Daily drinking was considered steady. Drinkers who did not fit into the classification because of variation in drinking habits were excluded. The ethnic and social background of the study population was rather homogeneous, thus decreasing the likelihood of confounding, that is interference due to other explaining factors. However, some major confounders were likely to remain, and we do not know how much influence on the mortality percentages these might have had. Smoking was one of those potential major confounders, although unknown at that time. Later, in 1938, Pearl was the first to show that also smoking increased mortality. Pearl was ahead of his time. The importance of his work remained nearly forgotten for more than 50 years. His main point has not always made clear. In a book published as recently as 2013, the survival curve for all moderate drinkers was contrasted to that of abstainers, thus concealing the difference between occasional and steady moderate drinkers. Only in the late 1970's was new important information on drinking habits and health obtained, most likely by lucky accident.

After World War II, a great increase in heart disease mortality was noted. Several studies were designed to investigate its causes. The major suspects were dietary habits (especially fat intake), smoking, lack of exercise and high blood pressure. Alcohol intake was included among the data collected, probably because it constituted one part of dietary energy. It may have been a surprise when several studies, starting from the late 1970's, found that moderate alcohol intake decreased the incidence of heart disease and mortality. The new research applied two useful statistical methods, unknown at the time Pearl conducted his studies. By statistical adjustment, a distinction could be made between the effect of

21

alcohol and known confounding factors (including other causal ones). Statistical theory provided tools to estimate the degree of accuracy of the study results. Mean and dispersion values of the outcome were statistically transformed into estimates of risk.

Risk is something that might occur in the future. You have an accident, or you find a wallet full of cash. You cannot be aware of what will happen in time, but you would like to minimize the risk of unpleasant incidents and perhaps maximize the occurrence of pleasant ones. How can you determine the magnitude of various risks? A common way is to use rules of thumb (scientists call these heuristics). But these are based on our past experience which often misleads. Better estimates can be derived from scientific studies. The studies are also based on past experience. However, the past experiences of thousands of persons can be added together. More effort is made to lessen random error and bias. The data are more rigorously ascertained. Pooled experience gives us the risk estimates, on two conditions. First, we presume that the future will be similar to the past. Secondly, we select a statistical model that seems to best correspond the underlying process. All models simplify the reality but some are useful in predicting the outcome. We presume that a study available to us at present is a sample of all possible populations, past, present and future combined. Then the incidence rate found in this study is the best estimate of the underlying true incidence rate. To get a rough idea of the degree of precision of the estimate, we can calculate confidence limits. This is done assuming that the incidence rate found in the study is free from bias, comes from a random sample of the infinite population and that in repeated samples from that population, the rates that will be found are distributed according to a known statistical law. Commonly, the 95 % confidence interval is calculated, abbreviated as 95 % CI. The true rate is commonly thought to be within the lower and upper limit of the interval in 95 cases out of 100 infinitely repeated samples. If this statistical reasoning is not clear, please do not worry, neither is it to all statisticians (Greenland & Poole 2013).

In practice, assumptions are less than fully met and confidence limits are best seen as a rough minimum estimate of the uncertainty. The more data we have, the more precise our estimates become. For this reason, similar studies are often combined in a process called meta-analysis. When comparing two groups, say abstainers and drinkers, the outcome, say mortality or the incidence of disease, is considered to differ between these groups if the significance is below 5 % ($p < 0.05$) and the 95 % CI does not include the number one. The next paragraph provides examples.

Relative risk values are simply reached by dividing the incidence in the group of interest by the risk in the comparison group. This is the standard way to report risks related to various health habits, laboratory values and environmental exposures. Now we are ready to see what modern studies tell us about alcohol intake and mortality. One large meta-analysis on mortality combined results from 31 studies (Ronksley et al. 2011). The findings were as follows (*Table 1*).

Table 1. Alcohol intake and relative risk of death from according to a meta-analysis

	Alcohol intake, g/day	Relative risk	95% Confidence interval
Non-drinkers	0	1	..
Lowest risk	2.5 - 15	0.83	0.80 - 0.86
Highest risk	60 or more	1.30	1.22 - 1.38

You see that alcohol intake is reported as grams per day. One 33 cl glass of beer, 12 cl of wine or 4 cl of hard liquor contains approximately 12 grams equalling approximately half an ounce of 100 % alcohol. This is what you might usually get when you order a drink in a bar. Gram (or some other weight unit) is the most unequivocal way to measure the amount of alcohol. It is better than the number of drinks because the size and alcohol content of a drink varies considerably. And weight does not depend on temperature as volume does.

To make comparisons easier, the amount of alcohol consumed is related to time, commonly over the whole time period in which the self-reports of drinking were recorded. Amount of intake is divided by the number of all days in the period, whether spent abstaining or drinking. For practical reasons, the time period cannot be too long. Otherwise forgetting undermines the recall of drinking. Therefore, intake data are usually ascertained from the past week, month, three months or some other short period. The shorter the period, the more the extremes are likely to be over-represented. However, it is tacitly assumed to represent the long-term average alcohol consumption.

Note that according to the above meta-analysis, abstainers had higher risk than moderate drinkers. Mortality for the latter was 14 - 20 % lower than among non-drinkers. The risk increase for the highest group is of higher magnitude than the respective decrease for the lowest risk group. If this kind of data is drawn into a curve, it will resemble a strongly flattened letter J, as in *Figure 1*.

The above meta-analysis did not report the intake level after which the mortality rate exceeds that of lifelong abstainers. Let us call this the risk level, or the level of risky drinking. Below it, drinking may provide more benefit than harm, above it the reverse is likely to hold true. One estimate for this level can be found in an earlier meta-analysis, based on the same studies with a few exceptions (Di Castelnuovo et al. 2006). More about it later in chapter 2.

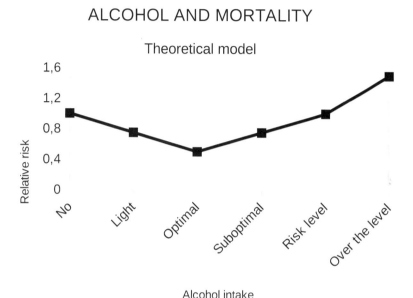

Figure 1. Alcohol and mortality - a theoretical model

Mortality is reasonably thoroughly studied. Less information is available about the incidence of diseases even if there are dozens of fairly large studies. These studies point out that the relation between alcohol intake and health is similarly flatly J-shaped as that for mortality. This is true for the incidence of hospital admissions, leaves of absence from work, work-disability pensions, physical fitness and self-reported health status. The decreased incidence among moderate drinkers, compared with that among abstainers, is true for coronary heart disease, stroke, diabetes, dementia and gallstones.

There is more in drinking than the average. Alcohol intake varies over time. It is like beating the drum. The long-term average number of beats is not the music. We hear also the rhythm of beating and the volume of sound. From the health point of view, alcohol intake is similar. The relevant features are the long-term average number of drinks, the rhythm of imbibing drinks and the speed of drinking, the latter because it is the cause of alcohol level changes in the body. Next let us see what we know about the rhythm of drinking. Later in Part II we will talk about speed of drinking, blood alcohol levels and intoxication.

Drinking rhythm and health

To separate the effects of the amount (average number of drinks) and the rhythm is not easy if we want very detailed information. Often we have to be satisfied with simplifying questions to map out the variability, just like Raymond Pearl did in his classic study on mortality.

A common way is to ask separately about light and heavy drinking occasions. Questions about the latter may focus either on occasions with intoxication or on those exceeding a certain number of drinks. Both ways have some strengths and some weaknesses. It is easier to remember the frequency of intoxication. However, what people consider as intoxication

27

varies. The definition of a heavy drinking occasion varies also. It can be more than two drinks, seven drinks or something else. Often it is five drinks or more. The number of drinks does not tell anything about the time span spent in consuming the drinks. Five drinks taken rapidly in may lead to clear intoxication but the same number hardly has any material effect during a three-hour dinner. One man's binge is another man's gourmet meal. Despite these caveats, we can say something about the effects of drinking rhythm.

After adjusting for the average long-term alcohol intake, heavy drinking occasions may increase the risk of suboptimal self-reported health, coronary heart disease, stroke, depression and injury. Findings, however, are not consistent. Some studies have not found any additional effect. To my knowledge, only one study has described the effects of drinking rhythm in great detail. The outcome was the incidence of coronary heart disease (McElduff & Dobson, 1997). In this Australian case-control study, one drink contained 10 g of alcohol. Highest risk was found among men who consumed 90 g or more either every day or during one or two days every week. Lowest risk was found among those men who consumed less but rather frequently - 30 to 60 g/day during 3 to 6 days a week. Their risk was about half of that among lifelong abstainers (*Table 2*). The relative risks were adjusted for age, smoking and previous major disease. There were 11,511 cases with disease and 6,077 control persons. Although the study group was very large, many subgroups remained small. Several risk estimates were imprecise because of too wide confidence intervals. Significance of the relative risk estimates must be taken with a pinch of salt because the study did not say whether correction for multiple testing was applied or not. The table illustrates what kind of data we would like to have to separate the effects of amount and rhythm. Very large study populations would be needed to obtain more precise risk estimates if drinking patterns are divided into very detailed categories. For more general groupings, some new findings have recently emerged.

Self-rated health is simply how people respond when asked whether they think that their health is very good, rather good, average, rather poor or very poor. This 5-point scale predicts mortality rather well. A large Swedish study between the years 2002-2014 divided drinking trajectories into five groups. Compared with stable moderate drinkers, all other trajectories were associated with poor self-rated health. The occurrence of poor health was for stable non-drinkers 2.35-fold, for unstable non-drinkers 2.58-fold, for former drinkers 2.81-fold, and for stable heavy drinkers 2.16-fold (Gémes et al 2019). An English study among the aged found that never-drinkers and ex-drinkers had more often poor self-rated health that current drinkers. The latter were divided into seven groups on the basis of the amount and rhythm of drinking. Compared with the occasional light drinkers, heavy frequent drinkers (amount men <21, women <14 British units per week almost every day) had fewer people with poor self-rated health. The other drinker groups did not differ from the comparison group

(Frisher et al. 2015).

Table 2. Number of 10 g drinks, number of drinking days and the relative risk of coronary heart disease (lifelong abstainers = 1).

Number of drinking days in a week

Drinks/day

	< 1	1 - 2	3 - 4	5 - 6	7
Men					
1 - 2	0.99	0.93	0.75	0.36	1.20
3 - 4	**0.44**	0.91	**0.56**	**0.46**	0.87
5 - 8	1.13	1.00	**0.46**	**0.50**	0.83
9 or more	0.99	**2.62**	1.93	2.22	**2.40**
Women					
1 - 2	0.76	0.69	**0.39**	0.52	0.95
3 - 4	1.18	0.53	0.77	1.41	0.40
5 or more	1.29	2.03	1.28	0.32	2.82

Risk ratios in bold are statistically significant ($p < 0.05$). Confidence intervals can be found in the original report. McElduff & Dobson 1997.

30

We can, however, construct theoretical models to illustrate the effects of stable and irregular drinking on health. Let us assume that we compare a stable pattern, say an equal amount of alcohol all seven days a week, and an irregular pattern, say four days of abstinence and three drinking days every week. And assume that the effect is directly related to the daily amount. For example, irregular drinkers have the same risk than abstainers on the days of their sobriety and the same risk on drinking days as steady drinkers would have if the latter imbibed the amount the former do. This is the simplest assumption we can arrive at. *Figure 2* shows what we might see given these assumptions. Note that steady intake (the long black continuous curve) has more beneficial risk ratios at the moderate intake level than does irregular intake (the short grey dashed curve). Actual relations are most likely to be more complicated and more difficult to model. Alcoholics drink not only much but also with accelerated rhythm and speed. It is a 7/24 hobby. They have much higher mortality than other drinkers. More about this later in Part VII.

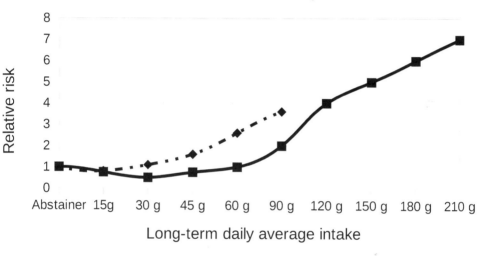

Figure 2. Alcohol and relative risk: regular 7/7 days a week (black curve) and irregular 3/7 days a week rhythm (grey curve)days a week rhythm (grey curve)

3 What is the risk level of alcohol intake? - More indulgent than you have been told

Virtue does not lie in following guidelines but in a judicious setting of your own rules.

Once upon a time, the ministry of health in a far-away country wanted to recruit an expert to ascertain the risk level of alcohol intake. A headhunter asked the first applicant: "In your view, what is the real risk level?". The applicant said: "Zero. It is clear that all alcohol intake is bad for the health. It brings about many diseases and leads into alcoholism." The headhunter responded: "This might be so but it is politically impossible. We cannot call for prohibition again." The second applicant pondered the same question a long time and said: "A difficult question but the medical profession knows best. Therefore, the risk level is as much as your doctor drinks." "Impossible", said the headhunter, "we cannot allow the population consume such huge amounts." The third applicant got the job. The winning answer was: "How much do you want it to be?"

Many official and professional groups have published guidelines on the risky levels of drinking. Likewise, recommended levels or safe levels have been presented. These all are guesstimates and underestimates. They are guided more by what is thought to be politically correct than by scientific

33

evidence. They differ from each other and seem to be too low, but how much too low is difficult to say. There is no consensus and no such can be reached on the basis of scientific evidence.

It is important to understand what the concepts *risk level* and *safe level* mean. They are population concepts, denoting to what is the average risk in a population group exposed to some substance, compared with an unexposed group. They do not determine the fate for any certain individual. There is no 100 % guarantee that you will avoid something bad or gain something good. Safe level also supposes that instructions and safeguards have been properly followed. As to alcoholic beverages, moderation is the safe way.

The risk level of alcohol intake is hard to estimate. Risk levels vary depending on the outcome we are interested in. Epidemiologic studies have shown that drinking can increase the risk of the onset some diseases, decrease that of some others and have no influence on the rest. The same goes for the risk of death. So what are the most relevant target outcomes? The most comprehensive ones. These are the all-cause (aka total) mortality and suboptimal health. Suboptimal health can be measured either as the onset of any disease or self-reported poor health. There are only a few studies of the latter two. The onset of disease and death can also sometimes be combined to the most comprehensive outcome. Alas, it is usually not easy because the incidence (onset) of many diseases can not be exactly ascertained, in contrast to the moment of death.

All-cause mortality has been studied extensively.

34

Therefore, it is best to focus on it when trying to calculate the risk level of alcohol intake. What is the best comparison group? Obviously those who have never used alcohol. Thus, let us try to find out the drinking level where the risk of death meets that of lifelong abstainers.

Let us first try to find out the most likely estimate for the risk level (known as point-estimate in scientific literature). No meta-analysis has reported a best estimate of the above risk level in plain numbers. The figure 4A in the meta-analysis by Dr. Di Castelnuovo and his coworkers, however, has the curve we need. With the help of the naked eye and measuring tools we can see that the risk level is more or less 33 g/day (Di Castelnuovo et al. 2011). This underestimates the risk level because of three reasons. First, at least two studies were excluded. Of these, the very important one is the *American Cancer Society Study, Cancer Prevention Study II* (Thun et al. 1997). This study found that even in the highest intake group, consuming 72 g/day or more, the risk of death was lower than among lifelong abstainers. The relative risk of death was just a little below one. For men the relative risk was 0.96 (95 % CI 0.93 - 1.00) and for women 0.98 (95 % CI 0.89 - 1.07). So we are on the safe side if we make the conservative assumption that the aforementioned 72 g/day is the risk level. These findings were based on the experience of 490,000 persons. To this we can add the 37,000 persons from an Australian study with results closely similar to that of the American one (Baglietto et al. 2006). The meta-analysis estimate was based on the experience of approximately one million persons (Di Castelnuovo et al. 2006). Since the number of person-years were not reported, we have no better way than to use the number of persons in calculating the weighted average. The rough calculation yields 46 g/day for the best risk level estimate. Respective calculations for men and women separately can only be made with all abstainers as the comparison group. In this comparison, the risk level for men is 50 g/day and for women 47 g/day. This was the result in the first edition of this book. A more recent meta-analysis consisted of about 2.5 million persons. It did not include the aforementioned *American Cancer Society Study* (Thun et al. 1997) but there were data from two large unpublished studies. It found that the risk level was approximately 75 g/day for men and 50 g/day for women (Wang et al. 2014). Figure 3 in this meta-analysis suggests that the lower 95 % confidence limit for men is approximately 30 g/day, while the upper confidence limit remains unknown because even at the level of 80 g/day, the heaviest level available, the risk does not reach that of abstainers. For women the limits are 30-60 g/day. The above estimates are the best we have but remain unsatisfactory. Ideally, all the available studies should be combined, but this is beyond the scope of the present book.

A few efforts have been made to combine the incidence (onset) of some diseases and death to obtain estimates on life span changes due to certain risk factors or diseases. A major study estimated the effect of five healthy lifestyles on life spans in the US Population 50 years of age. One of these lifestyles was moderate alcohol intake (men 5-30 g/day; women 5-15 g/day). The outcome was life expectancy free of cardiovascular disease, cancer and type2 diabetes. Compared with men with four healthy lifestyles (no smoking, high physical activity, ideal body mass index and healthy diet), those who were also drinking moderately had 0.8 years longer life expectancy. The respective increase for women was 3 years (Li et al. 2020).

Life span calculations are captivatingly easy to grasp but also easy to misunderstand. They apply to certain defined times and populations. They are not the fate for an individual, and not universal constants, although some scientific papers and the media may foist this false idea. Incidences of disease and death (morbidity and mortality) are considered to have a more general validity.

All the above estimates of risk levels are not very accurate for two reasons. One pertains to epidemiologic cohort studies in general. Even if these studies do their best to eliminate (by statistical adjusting) the influence of other factors (confounders), there always remains the possibility that some confounders have not been controlled for, have not been measured or remain unknown. A better way to control for confounding would be to do randomized trials. Alas, there are no such studies on alcohol and all-cause mortality. However, some randomized evidence is available for intermediate causes of end outcomes. More about these later.

The second reason is the poor quality of information on

37

alcohol intake. Self-reports are notoriously unreliable.[3] Most people underestimate their alcohol intake. The degree of underestimation varies but usually the actual intake is on average 2- to 3-fold compared with the reported one (Alanko 1984, Knibbe & Bloomfield 2001, Rossow et al. 2014). This has been found when the average reported alcohol intake in representative random samples of population has been compared with the registered alcohol sales in the same population. Rigorous diary-keeping in small study groups have shown slightly less underestimation than questionnaires. Thus, the actual risk level is likely to be higher than what the face value findings tell us. Corrected for under-reporting, the risk levels will sound high to you, but please note two things. First, the above correction for underestimation relies on crude averages of underestimation. Some studies suggest higher coefficients of correction. For example, the actual per capita intake in France has been found to be 5-fold compared with the

---

[3]   Four alcohol scientists wanted to enliven their small WHO meeting in Phoenix by admiring the Grand Canyon from the air. The small plane pilot asked about their exact body weights. Then the respondents were led to a set of scales and the truth was revealed. Three of the scientists had underreported their weight by about 22 pounds (*A book of letters for Robin Room: celebrating fifty years of research and service.* No publication date nor place. Available also at https://dpmp.unsw.edu.au/resource/room [accessed December 19, 2014]).

survey self-reports (Rey et al. 2010). Secondly, careful participant observations have found that many alcoholics consume much more, typically between 350 to 470 g/day (Poikolainen 1977, p.122). In some old experiments, not very ethical according to current standards, alcoholics consumed voluntarily up to 400 g of alcohol per day and would have taken more in the interest of advancing science, were not the researchers against their noble offers (Mendelson & La Dou 1964).

Another problem is that self-reports on alcohol intake pertain to a short period before the date of examination. Even if the recall period is longer, say six months or more, self- reports are more influenced by recently consumed amounts rather than the actual long-term average. The past is viewed through the spectacles of the present. Some persons are likely to have had more to drink than what is their long-term average, and some less. This would inflate the risk level, but how much, we have no idea.

One hidden assumption in epidemiologic studies is that the risk factors remain constantly at the same level. In this case ascertainment of the level of exposure during a short period is a good indicator of the overall exposure. In some cases this is a reasonable assumption. For example, the number of cigarettes smoked daily tends to be about the same among regular smokers. In the case of alcohol intake there is much more variability. Actual drinking patterns and consumed amounts may change over time. Little is known about the effects

39

patterns and changes have on health. Luckily, many study groups consist mainly of middle-aged or older persons, and changes in these groups are smaller than among young adults. Moreover, they provide some evidence. An Australian study where alcohol intake was interviewed for 10-year periods found that association between all-cause mortality intake was J-shaped for all the three variables: lifetime, current and maximum past consumption. Considering lifetime intake, men drinking less than 40 g/day and women 10 g/day had lower mortality than those consuming more (Jayasekara et al. 2015). Ex-drinkers in good health at the baseline examination have higher risk of death than their lightly drinking peers in follow-up studies (Poikolainen 2016b). Similar findings pertaining to cardiovascular diseases will be presented in the next chapter.

To sum up, it is really hard to find where the risk level for all-cause mortality lies. We can be sure that it must be much higher than the ridiculously low 10-20 g/day that the professional or official guidelines claim. Fake truths! Maybe the level is 50, 75, 100 g/day or even higher. I know eminent scientists who have refused to participate in guideline committees because setting reliable limits is in their view impossible. Nevertheless, guidelines are published. And the newer the guidelines, the lower is the risk level. The latest British guidelines recommend a maximum of 16 g of alcohol (1.25 drinks) per day. The authors of this recommendation must be worried about the health of Queen Elizabeth II. Her Majesty has been said to enjoy four drinks a day - a cocktail and a glass

40

of wine for lunch, a dry martini and a glass of champagne for dinner.[4]

Despite the inherent uncertainty, all guidelines are marketed as definite ones. Why? Otherwise, brief interventions to reduce alcohol intake would be impossible. Instead of a risk level guideline, total abstinence would be the advice. But demanding prohibition would prove to be unacceptable to the general public and thus an intractable policy. Historical experience is too well known. Even the anti-alcohol academics understand this. These experts seem to like the paternalistic, messianic role of defining what is in their view in the best interests of the lay people. It has been argued that many academics "implicitly regard the normative function of their profession as more important than commitment to scientific certainty." (Yeomans 2013). Already Plato in his *Republic* (380 BC) thought that common people must be protected from thruths by noble lies.[5] Not surprisingly, George Bernard Shaw (1856 ~ 1950) quipped: every profession is a conspiracy against the common man.

---

[4]   http://google.com/newsstand/s/CBIwzP-M0DU

[5]   "Whereas the lie in words is in certain cases useful and not hateful; ... when those whom we call our friends in a fit of madness or illusion are going to do some harm, then it is useful and is a sort of medicine or preventive"

41

Make your own rules

I do not oppose guidelines in general. But guidelines for the general public should be simple, valid, easy to apply, and bring about a substantial benefit to those following the advice. Guidelines based on inaccurate or weakly validated evidence can do more harm than good. When the evidence is poor and individual variation great it is better to make one's own rules, applying the available evidence carefully. Some controversy prevails as to moderate alcohol intake is really beneficial or not. It might seem to some that in this case it is best to apply a precautionary principle: to abstain totally from alcohol, no drink, no harm. But if moderation is beneficial, abstainers are exposed to some health risk. For those who want to judge the evidence on this, chapter 4 discusses the scientific debate on this subject.

My view holds that according to the current best evidence the beneficial effects of moderate intake are real. In want of more accurate evidence, it seems prudent to accept the largest meta-analysis available with the best estimate for the risk level with respect to mortality of approximately 75 g/day for men and 50 g/day for women. The optimal level from the point of survival is probably about half the risk level, because the risk curve is rather symmetric at low consumption levels. Taking into account the underestimation of alcohol intake it seems that these estimates are lower than the actual risk levels and thus err on the safe side.

More sensible than pondering where the risk limit lies in

adopting some judicious habits. Rhythm and drinking speed play a major role. *Fruens tardius*. Drink slowly and enjoy, preferably around evening meals. Adjust your drinking so that you sleep well and feel good in the mornings. Avoid drinking elevating your blood pressure and watch your body weight.

The textbooks tell that the energy value of one gram of alcohol is 7 kcal. It is lower than the 9 kcal for fat but higher than 4 kcal for carbohydrates or proteins. However, intestinal bacteria will consume a good deal of all alcohol before it enters your metabolic system. One study on six subjects found that 80 %, not 100 %, of the energy from alcohol was in fact used for metabolism (Suter et al. 1994). Thus, the energy from 1 g of alcohol available for your body is likely to be about 5.6 kcal, lower than what the textbooks report. Alcohol does not add to your weight if you do not take in more calories than you burn.

Moral implications of risk

There is also a moral lesson. Risk is likelihood, not fate. Risk estimates suggest the likelihood of something that may happen in future, but do not prove that it will. Moreover, the comparison groups used in relative risk calculations are also at risk, even if their risk is lower than those having higher risk. Lifelong abstainers are not immune to accidents, cancer or liver cirrhosis.

Would you consider a person who drinks more than at a certain risk level, or somebody who abstains totally from drinking, morally bad? It is questionable to attach moral values

43

to risk estimates. Moralistic views equate risk behavior and getting a disease. This leads to holding people with risky behaviors responsible for the disease if they get it, and to demands that the cost of any treatment should be paid by the person at risk (Heyman 2010). This is unfair, because no one can be 100 percent certain of avoiding the occurrence of some disease by sidestepping a risk behavior. Risk estimates do not dictate the future. For example, a plausible estimate of coronary heart disease risk for lifelong abstainers, in relation to moderate drinkers, would be 1.25. Applying the formula (RR - 1)/RR, where RR is the risk ratio (relative risk), shows that in this case the lack of alcohol intake explains 20 percent of the incidence of coronary heart disease among abstainers. Other causal factors are needed to explain the rest of the risk. In the same way, if the relative risk for lung cancer is 10 among regular smokers, smoking explains 90 percent of the incidence among these, not 100 percent. Other factors than the risk factor under study play a role in causation. Some people differ from the average in ways that give reasons for deviant practices. They might have some important economic, hedonistic, ideological, religious or health reasons for their behavior. Health is an important value in general, but there are other values, as well.

Putting the blame on somebody who cannot control the future is counterproductive. It is common that diseases have several known and also unknown risk factors and we can control only one part of these to some extent. The several risk factors for some major alcohol-related diseases will be reviewed in Part V.

45

4 The good effects of moderation are real - despite what the anti-alcohol academics say

The scientific evidence strongly supports the positive effects of moderation. The anti-alcohol academics cannot swallow this unpalatable truth.

In epidemiologic studies, moderate alcohol intake has been found to decrease the risk of coronary heart disease, stroke related to blood clots, dementia and adult-type diabetes. These diseases are all more or less related to blood vessels. Findings about these beneficial effects of alcohol intake are often opposed by arguing that these findings are not absolutely certain. The opponents do not, on the other hand, criticise findings that alcohol intake has harmful effects, even if such findings in both directions have been made in the same study by the same methods.

I call these opponents anti-alcohol academics since most of them are have a university education. They tend to believe that all alcohol use harms and they manipulate scientific methods to produce evidence in support of their views. When meeting them, they seemed courteous, nice and clever people. Some perhaps abstain, most like to drink and party. It seems that they believe to be immune to the harms of alcohol and above the evidence that disputes their belief. I am not trying to convince them. The arguments below are for those open to

46

consider all facts.

The lower heart disease risk among moderate drinkers compared with abstainers is attributed by the anti-alcohol academics in denial to unknown differences between the two groups, abstainers having some hidden unhealthy factors. If this is true, higher risk of death would be expected to be found not only from cancer but also from heart disease among drinkers. However, there are studies where moderate alcohol intake decreases the heart death risk but increases monotonically the breast cancer risk without any evidence of a J-shape. The largest one is the Nurses' Health Study, initially including 121,700 women. Reduced all-cause death rates were found among moderate drinkers (Colditz et al. 1997; Baer et al. 2011). Of the nurses, 34 % abstained from alcohol (Baer et al. 2011).

The anti-alcohol academics take the harmful effects for granted. This is patently not true, science holds no absolute certainties. In Berthold Brecht's play *Galileo*, the protagonist says that the goal of science is not to open the door to endless wisdom but set limits to endless erring. That is the very point. The philosophical foundations of this view have been presented lucidly by Ronald Giere in his book *Scientific Perspectivism* (Giere 2006). This line of scientific realism points out that scientific truths are not absolute or final. They simply are our best knowledge at present, seen from the perspective of the field of study in question. Sometimes, when we are lucky, they are models that well explain and allow us to modify what is

47

happening with high enough accuracy to produce consistent results. This works as long as other factors remain constant or do not alter too much to interfere with the application of our theoretical models. And when models perform well they are often called the laws of nature.

Scientific perspectivism differs from objectivistic realism. The latter believes in final truths. In this it is similar to religious dogmatism. It is a popular view because it props up beliefs in experts' infallibility and lessens the need for independent thinking. Scientific perspectivism differs also from constructivism, although unknown things may leave room for doubt and constructivistic ideas. These maintain that there are only various views and theories, but no best option among the views. At best, there might be a general consensus on something even if it cannot be proven to be the best explanation. We'll meet constructivism again in Part VI that deals with alcoholism. Now we will discuss the strength of the evidence for the beneficial effects of alcohol intake.

Lifelong abstainers are the best comparison group when the effects of alcohol intake on health are under study. However, some British researchers oppose this by saying that this group is small and deviates much from the general population. This is true for England and Wales, but not for the country where most major studies have been conducted. In the USA, abstainers comprise approximately one-third of the population and in some groups their number may reach 60 percent. Lifelong abstinence may be due to ethical or religious

48

motives, prevailing traditions or lack of interest. In Finland, no differences were found between lifelong abstainers and moderate drinkers that could explain differences in health (Poikolainen et al. 2005). The "sick lifelong abstainer" hypothesis is false.

While trying to tease out the effect of putative cause on the effect, epidemiologic follow-up studies can never control for all other confounding factors. Thus, the anti-alcohol academics can always imagine that there is some unknown factor that explains the health differences between lifelong abstainers and moderate drinkers. The onus of finding proof for this rests on them. I wish them luck. Finding evidence won't be easy. The differences found are so great and precise that any unknown factor must be a strong risk factor and be distributed very unevenly between lifelong abstainers and moderate drinkers.

The anti-alcohol academics argue that not all studies have found the J-shaped relation. This is understandable. If the follow-up period is short and the population cohort healthy at the onset of the study, cases of disease or death will not be sufficient to show statistically significant differences. If the sample under study does not comprise enough persons and enough diverse patterns of drinking, the J-shape cannot be observed. For example, if there are no moderate drinkers, a linear trend may be seen. If there are no heavy drinkers, you are likely to see a U-shape. Despite variations in the curvilinear relation between alcohol and all-cause mortality the beneficial

49

effect of light to moderate drinking can be found to be stable even when the heterogeneity between studies is taken into account (Gmel et al. 2003).

Meta-analysis is useful way to combine data from several studies to increase the precision of risk estimates. But it can be misused. Some anti-alcohol academics have applied unrealistic criteria in order to exclude important studies from their meta-analyses resulting in 'disappearance' of the beneficial effects of alcohol. Two tricks were used. First, excluded were studies where the criterion for lifelong abstaining was 'to have consumed not more that 12 alcoholic drinks (glasses) during lifetime' or a positive response 'never or almost never' or 'rarely/never' to the question 'How often do you drink?'. A few drinks during lifetime does not turn an abstainer into a regular moderate drinker. It does not wipe out the long-term effect of abstaining. Likewise, a few days of non-smoking does not wipe out the lung cancer risk for a regular smoker. Epidemiologic studies reveal the effects of long-term exposures. The second trick was to exclude a study showing the strongest beneficial effect of alcohol. No plausible reason was given; it was only said that the study was an outlier (Stockwell et al. 2016). The excluded study (Friesema et al. 2007) is an exceptionally good one. I have read it carefully. There is no reason to leave it out. The above kind of data abuse has ended up first with a midget meta-analysis that shows no statistical effect of alcohol on mortality. Even heavy drinking seemed harmless. I have earlier discussed this in more detail (Poikolainen 2008). The second attempt found that heaviest drinkers had lower mortality that moderate drinkers and not different from that of lifelong abstainers (Stockwell et al. 2016). Monkey business.

A real weakness of most studies is the lack of data on changes in alcohol intake people make over time. However, in some major studies these changes have been small or nonexistent because of the exclusion of people who had made stark changes in alcohol intake. When changes have been studied, the findings support the beneficial effect of moderate drinking. The incidence of cardiovascular diseases decreased 29 percent among those men who increased their alcohol intake over the follow-up period, from one drink or less per week to up to six drinks per week (Sesso et al. 2000). Women who increased their alcohol intake after the diagnosis of breast cancer lived longer than women who remained abstinent before and after the diagnosis (Newcomb et al. 2013). Moreover, starting drinking has a favorable and quitting drinking an adverse effect on fibrinogen, a cardiovascular risk factor (Okwuosa et al. 2013). And as noted above, ex-drinkers in good health at baseline examination have higher risk of death than their lightly drinking peers in follow-up studies (Poikolainen 2016b).

Randomized trials

The best comparisons of groups are randomized, that is, the study subjects are allocated into groups at random. Like in a

51

lottery. Randomization can make the distributions of all confounding factors, both known and unknown, similar in the groups, provided that the allocation process in unbiased and the size of the groups is large. If then one of the groups is given some treatment, such as moderate doses of alcohol and the other no alcohol, the resulting difference is most likely due to the alcohol dose, provided that everything else in the study is executed correctly. The randomized design is robust to possible biases due to confounding factors. However, to execute such studies flawlessly is not easy - just see how thick the guide books for randomized studies are.

Anti-alcohol academics like to call for randomized controlled trials. Other kinds of study design is not good enough for them on the relation between moderate intake and positive health, although for the adverse effects less rigorous designs are accepted. They are aware that such trials are very difficult to conduct. Large numbers of subjects would be required, the subjects would have to adhere to a strict regime of moderate drinking or abstinence, keeping everything else as constant as possible for ten years or more. But when one such study was financed and begun the denialists succeeded in canceling its funding (Oppenheimer & Bayer 2019). The main pretext was that cancer was not among the outcomes and that would not even have been feasible.

It seems to be unethical to ask people to abstain such a long time since we have strong evidence for the health benefits of moderate drinking. The responsibility of carrying out such

52

trials must rest on the anti-alcohol academics if they are not satisfied with the present evidence. Anti-alcohol academics who only accept evidence from randomized controlled trials should also conclude that no firm evidence has been presented showing that alcohol causes liver cirrhosis, smoking causes lung cancer, and obesity increases the risk of heart disease as well as many other diseases. Many would like this kind of utopian world.

As long as we do not have randomized trials on final outcomes, such as the onset of disease or death, it is more sensible to trust the evidence provided by observational epidemiology than to remain ignorant. If we had randomized studies, we must remember that these kind of studies on other questions have shown contradictory results, have often been valid only for selected population groups and have often been in agreement with observational studies.

While we do not have randomized trials on final outcomes, we do have evidence on the biological mechanisms playing a role in mediating the effects of alcohol on health. The risk of coronary heart disease and stroke is increased when arteries narrow and harden. This is brought about partly by cholesterol that is transported to the blood vessel walls by the 'bad' low-density lipoprotein (LDL) cholesterol. The 'good' high-density lipoprotein (HDL) cholesterol opposes this process by transporting cholesterol away from the walls. Randomized experiments have shown that alcohol intake increases the HDL levels. One meta-analysis found that an

53

alcohol dose of 30 g/day increased HDL approximately 8.3 percent (Rimm et al. 1999). This was confirmed in a later meta-analysis (Brien et al. 2011). The latter meta-analysis found that the higher the intake, the higher also the resulting increase in HDL. The latter meta-analysis also confirmed the beneficial effects on fibrinogen that opposes the formation of blood clots as well as on adiponectin, related both to coronary heart disease and diabetes. These beneficial effects were observed already among young adults (Brien et al. 2011). Therefore, we can refute the anti-alcohol academics' claim that the beneficial effects would be restricted to middle-aged or older people.

Recently, there has been some controversy about the protective effect of HDL cholesterol on CHD while LDL-cholesterol is clearly a major risk factor for CHD. The effect of alcohol on LDL is variable, but many studies (Brinton 2010), including randomized crossover trials (Baer et al. 2002, van der Gaag et al. 2000, Beulens et al. 2007), have found marked decreases. Moreover, a large Mendelian analysis has found that alcohol intake decreases LDL cholesterol (Tabara et al. 2016).

A 2-year long randomized trial showed that a daily amount of red wine (15 cl) had a beneficial effect on several CHD risk factors among well-controlled type 2 diabetics (Gepner et al. 2015). Among 224 patients red wine significantly increased high-density lipoprotein cholesterol (HDL-C) and apolipoprotein(a)1, while decreasing the total cholesterol-HDL-C ratio. Slow ethanol metabolizers (alcohol dehydrogenase alleles [ADH1B*1] carriers) significantly benefited from the effect of wine on glycemic control (fasting plasma glucose, homeostatic model assessment of insulin resistance, and hemoglobin A1c) compared with fast ethanol metabolizers (persons homozygous for ADH1B*2). No material harmful effects were found in blood pressure, adiposity, liver function, drug therapy, symptoms, or quality of life. Sleep quality improved in both red and white wine groups compared with the water group.

Genetic studies

Genes play an important role in many diseases. Most epidemiologic studies do not control for genetic makeup. Twin studies are an exception. Identical (monozygotic) twins both have the same genes, while dizygotic twins share 50 % of the genes. In a co-twin study, an inverse overall and within-pair relation between alcohol intake and Coronary heart disease (CHD) mortality risk was found. The higher the alcohol intake, the lower the CHD mortality. This was independent of genetic makeup, early life environment, adulthood experience and several other risk factors (Dai et al. 2015). This is strong evidence for the beneficial effect of alcohol on CHD.

Randomization can be mimicked if some factor randomly divides people into those who shun alcohol and those who are more likely to drink. If the factors are genes, this is often called Mendelian randomization. Despite random allocation of genes, Mendelian studies have some serious pitfalls (Ebrahim and

Davey Smith 2008).

There are a few hundred genes and thousands of gene variants involved in the effects of alcohol in the body. Of these, those determining the production of the enzymes taking part in the oxidation of alcohol have been of much interest. Ethyl alcohol is transformed into acetaldehyde by alcohol dehydrogenase (ADH) enzymes and acetaldehyde into acetic acid by acetaldehyde dehydrogenase (ALDH) enzymes. There are several different forms of both these two enzymes. Acetaldehyde is toxic but most people have gene variants that eliminate acetaldehyde very rapidly. A minority of people have more of this substance in the blood at any given moment, enough to cause unpleasant alcohol-induced symptoms. This is more common among Oriental people than among others. Persons with high acetaldehyde levels are likely to avoid alcohol completely or drink only a little, and shun intoxication. The studies have shown that genetic makeup has some influence on alcohol consumption. Moderate drinkers who are homozygous for the slow-oxidizing ADH3 variant have been shown to have substantially lower risk for myocardial infarction than those having the fast-oxidizing variant compared with those with very low alcohol intake and the fast-oxidizing variant (Hines et al. 2001). Both abstinence or very low alcohol intake and fast oxidation thus seem to increase risk. Comparing groups that differ in the genetic makeup of ADH and ALDH is not Mendelian randomization if other factors also play a role in group formation. For example, one study in the medical journal Lancet focused on six population categories, grouped on the basis of genetic makeup, area of residence, and population mean alcohol intake among the Chinese. The latter grouping factors were determined by the researchers, not by random distribution. The outcome was cardiovascular disease risk. The gene forms were ALDH2 (rs671) and ADH1B (rs1229984). The variants of these genes divide individuals into AA, AG or GG types (Millwood et al. 2019). The relation between alcohol intake and incidence of CHD and stroke was studied both using the above grouping and in a more conventional grouping of various consumption levels, never-drinkers and ex-drinkers. The first comparison misleads us to think that there was a Mendelian randomization and that its results refute the findings on protective effects from other studies.

If you dig deep enough into the web supplement an actual Mendelian analysis can be found. I shall focus on the ALDH2, since it has more influence on alcohol intake and on men, and since women consumed only minuscule amounts of alcohol. Of the three groups, AA had the lowest, AG intermediate and GG the highest mean alcohol intake. The respective self-reported mean values were 3, 37 and 157 grams of alcohol per week. Between the three groups there was no statistically significant difference in myocardial infarction or total CHD incidence (webfigure 6). However, the relationship was U-shaped, the AG group having the lowest CHD risk, suggesting that a larger data set could reveal significant differences. The age- and area-adjusted point-estimate of the risk ratio for total stroke in the GG group was 1.19, significantly higher but does not greatly differ from that for the AG group (webtable 18). This Mendelian comparison suggests that alcohol intake has no effect on CHD and high intake is related to a small increased stroke risk among the Chinese studied.

A common drawback in studies on the genetic variation in ADH and ALDH is that they do not control for drinking patterns. Differences in acetaldehyde levels, known to cause disturbing alcohol-induced symptoms, influence binge drinking and intoxication (Holmes et al. 2014). The latter is an important causal factor in alcohol-related cardiovascular diseases. Mendelian analyses of ADH and ALDH cannot account for this.

Animal experiments

Last and perhaps not least evidence comes from animal experiments. In Canada, the relation between alcohol consumption and life-span was studied in mice. Each group was given a constant daily amount of alcohol. Shortest life-span was among those with the highest dose, corresponding to a human intake of about 10 - 11 drinks daily. Longest life-span was related to a dose corresponding to a human intake of about 6 - 7 drinks daily. Abstinent mice had shorter life-span than the latter group (Schmidt et al. 1987). Similar findings have been found in Germany and Finland in the rat. The strain preferring alcohol had longer life-span than the rats shunning alcohol

(Sarviharju et al. 2004).

Blood pressure

Another potentially harmful effect is the increase in blood pressure. Pressure does not seem to increase if the intake is stable and remains below the level of 30 - 60 g/day (27). Hypertension is likely above this level if you do not have the constitution of Sir Winston Churchill. His blood pressure level was alleged to be 140/80 mmHg well into his eighties in spite of a respectable alcohol intake, perhaps partly to alleviate his depression.[6] At present we have potent drugs to decrease blood pressure. One study suggests that anti-hypertensive drugs can oppose and perhaps prevent the alcohol-induced increase in blood pressure (Wakabayashi 2010).

To sum up, the weight of the evidence shows that moderate drinking is better than abstaining and heavy drinking is worse than abstaining. There is a good deal of uncertainty in the risk estimates on alcohol intake and health. Nevertheless, this is better than no evidence at all because it at least helps to limit error. Success is more likely if you follow what is a balanced view on all evidence rather than the guidelines laid down by well-meaning anti-alcohol academics.

---

[6]   www.winstonchurchill.org

II

UNDER THE INFLUENCE - BLOOD ALCOHOL AND ACUTE EFFECTS

60

In addition to the quantity and rhythm of alcohol intake, also the speed of change in blood alcohol levels plays a major role in determining the effects of drink, especially the short-term ones generally known as being under the influence, intoxication, drunkenness and hangover. I have seen newspaper articles relating that the driver was intoxicated at the level of 0.02 %. You might reach this blood alcohol level after drinking a teacup of beer. Is this a case of serious drunkenness?

Drunkenness is both literally and figuratively a fuzzy concept. Where does it begin and where does it turn into poisoning? There are no clear limits, only changes in degrees. The short-time effect is the third factor, like the force of beating the drum or the resulting volume of sound. It also varies. The brain adapts to and compensates for all or part of the changes brought about by alcohol, both the good and the bad. Experimental studies help us to avoid the bad short-term effects and favor the pleasant ones.

61

5 The rise and fall of blood alcohol

What goes up must come down.

There is a close correlation between blood alcohol levels and the acute effects of alcohol. It is not, however, perfect or linear. The correlation is due to the fact that (ethyl) alcohol is a small molecule and soon becomes evenly distributed in the body water after it has traveled from the mouth to the stomach, then absorbed from the gut and carried by blood circulation to the tissues. The main part of acute effects are those taking place in the brain. We obtain rough estimates of the effects on the body from blood alcohol measurements.

There are several different conventions in use to report blood alcohol concentration (BAC). In this book I employ that used in Australia, Canada and the USA. These countries report concentrations by weight per volume, e.g. mg per 100 ml, often abbreviated to mg% or simply %. [7]

---

[7]   Most Central European countries also express the concentration in weight per volume. The unit, however, is pro mille (per thousand), e.g. g/L. Great Britain prefers basis points, that is weight per 10,000, e.g. 100 mg/L. One pro mille is 10 basis points or 0.1 %. Germany and the Nordic countries report in pro mille units, but these are by weight per weight, e.g. g/kg, often expressed as o/oo. Volume varies by

62

Laboratory research relies mostly on a very simple, general, exaggerated and non-natural design, because it is easy and it will intensify the acute effects of alcohol. After fasting overnight, volunteers rapidly drink a large dose of some alcoholic beverage next morning, with no more alcohol after that. Alcoholics may start their day like this, but they will not stop there.

Blood alcohol concentration is measured repeatedly in short intervals. Typically, you first see a steep rise of BAC (it is called the absorptive phase), the peak is reached, and finally there is a slower and approximately linear decrease of BAC (surprise, it is termed the post-absorptive phase). In one experiment, for example, after a dose of 2.26 oz (64 g) of alcohol mixed with 4 oz (116 ml) of water, the peak level of 0.12 % was reached in an hour and zero level came after seven more hours (Haggard et al. 1941).

Alcohol molecules travel in an instant from the mouth to the stomach without any substantial effects. The small intestine is the part of the tube where the molecules are absorbed into blood and then carried by circulation to all tissues containing water, meaning almost everywhere. Water constitutes about 50 - 75 % of the human body weight. The percentage depends mainly on sex, height and weight. Age is of no or little importance (Hume and Weyers 1971; Watson et al. 1981). For

temperature, weight does not. At normal laboratory temperature one pro mille weight per volume equals approximately 1.06 pro mille weight per weight.

example, the average water content of a man with a height of five feet 11 inches (180 cm) and weighing 187 lb (85 kg) is 57 % at the age of 20 years and 52 % at the age of 65 years. Sometimes it is claimed that old people are much more sensitive to the effects of alcohol because of their lower body water content. Not important from the scientific point of view.

If a man and a woman of equal height and weight consume the same dose of alcohol within the same short time period, the peak BAC will be higher and the decrease faster in the woman. This is simply because the average body water content is less in the woman. For example, given a five foot seven inch (170 cm) height, a 132 lb (60 kg) weight, and age of 20 years, the water content of our average woman would be 50 % and that of the man 65 %. However, the average man and the average woman are likely to differ both in height and weight, so we cannot expect large sex differences in the rise and fall of BAC.

Many factors influence the rise, peak and fall of BAC. Rise is slower in the evening than in the morning. It is also slower if the alcohol content of the beverage is lower, like in beer or wine, than in hard liquor, and if drinking is combined with eating rather than drinking between meals (Norberg et al. 2003). Examples of BAC curves are shown in *Figures 3 and 4*. For example, when the dose was 0.021 oz (0.6 g) of alcohol per kg of body weight, the average peak varied, according to a composite of studies, as follows (Leake and Silverman 1966 p. 54):

- Gin, vodka and whisky   0.10 %
- Fortified wine   0.06 %
- Natural wine   0.05 %
- Beer   0.04 %
- Natural wine and meal   0.03 %
- Beer and meal   0.02 %

Retarded rise and lower peak after a meal are partly due to the slower passage of alcohol from the stomach to the small intestine. Some unknown factors may also play a role. Without a meal, the first dose of spirits reaches the small intestine faster than other drinks. Further doses are slower because the emptying of the stomach becomes slower after the first dose (Kalant 2005).

The fall of BAC is practically linear after the peak if no more alcohol is consumed and the dose has not been exceptionally large. The rate of decrease is usually somewhere between 0.01 - 0.04 % but can be lower or higher. Heavy drinkers have faster rate than light or occasional drinkers.

The final portion disappears faster than the constant rate of linear decline. Not only the final part but the complete fall in heavy drinkers follows a more complex model than the linear one (Norberg et al. 2003; Kalant 2005; Wedell et al. 1991). The linear decline, based on the one water-compartment model, is actually an approximation that gives satisfactory results in most cases, but a more exact model has been defined (Wedell et al. 1991). Most experiments have been based on a small number

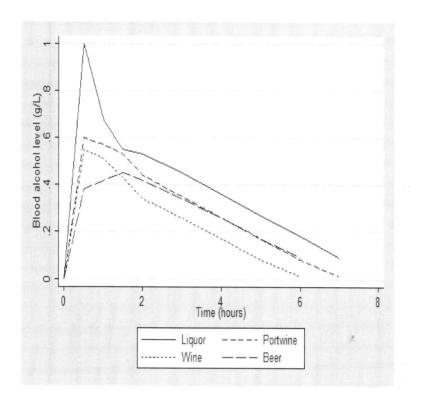

Figure 3. Blood alcohol curve variation after equal dose of alcohol as liquor, portwine, table wine or beer

of volunteers, say about a dozen. They may not represent well the average consumer. Larger studies show notable variation between the study subjects (Alha 1951; Jones 1984).

Alcohol is eliminated from the body mainly by oxidation in the liver. A small part of alcohol is eliminated in the expired air, sweat and urine. The elimination rate is constant during any drinking episode but varies between the episodes and people. The average rate is about 0.1 - 0.2 g per kg of body weight (Jones 1984; Loomis 1974). Having from half a drink to one drink per hour, say 6 - 12 g of alcohol, is not likely to increase BAC to any notable degree in the average adult.

Summing up, experimental evidence suggests that you can enhance the good and avoid the bad acute effects of alcohol by drinking slowly, preferring drinks with low alcohol percentage, eating something at the same time and drinking in the evenings. In everyday life, environment and the social situation are also of importance.

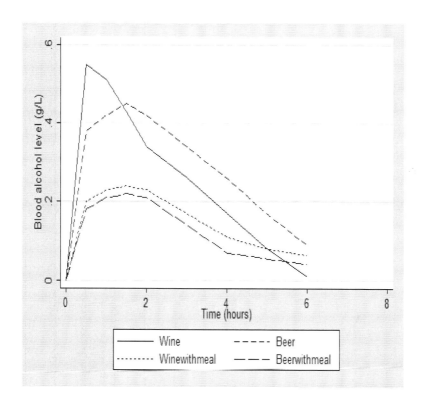

Figure 4. Blood alcohol curve variation after equal dose of alcohol as table wine or beer with or without food

6 The acute effects - Feeling good, feeling bad

The effects of alcohol in blood vary and can be regulated.

Blood alcohol is correlated with, but not directly related to, acute effects. Many factors intervene. The effects are stronger during the rise and the peak of blood alcohol than during the fall. Inexperienced users are subject to stronger effects than the seasoned ones. Very roughly, the correlation of blood alcohol and its effects can be as follows among inexperienced users.

Blood alcohol %	Effects
• 0.02 - 0.08	pleasure, relaxation, decreased attention, slower reaction time
• 0.08 - 0.2	weakened judgment, emotional lability, unsteady gait
• 0.2 - 0.3	unclear speech, malaise, vomiting
• 0.3 - 0.4	impaired memory, numbness, loss of consciousness
• 0.4 - 0.5	death from respiratory failure

Experienced users may show considerable tolerance to the effects of alcohol. Random road checks have revealed that some can drive a car satisfactorily when the alcohol content in

69

the blood is 0.3 - 0.4 %. A few have survived concentrations between 0.7 - 1.1 % with the help of treatment.

The lines between tipsiness, drunkenness, intoxication and poisoning are fuzzy as are those of hangover and withdrawal symptoms. To serve legal and medical needs, indicators that provide an approximate idea of the degree of performance impairment are needed. Blood alcohol level serves this purpose reasonably well. The bad effects

High and steeply rising blood alcohol can make you less intelligent, less conscientious or less good-natured, as well as more nervous or aggressive without any change in the core personality (Winograd et al. 2012). During the fall of blood alcohol you may feel tired, impassive, non-focused or depressed. If too much has been consumed, this can be followed by hangover symptoms like thirst, dry mouth, tremor, headache, anxiety, depression and many others.

Slower reaction time and unsteady coordination of movements increases the likelihood of every sort of accident. This is especially dangerous when operating a motor vehicle (more on this in chapter 19). The effects are influenced by the rate of the rise of blood alcohol, tolerance, personality traits and social situation. Despite tolerance, the risk of accident remains increased.

The good effects

Small amounts and slow drinking maximize the good effects. You may feel happy, hilarious, alert, energetic, active, sociable, eager and strong without any change in the core personality (Winograd et al. 2012; Brodsky and Peele 1999). Some of the good effects are due to the expectations based on beliefs. Cultural differences in beliefs and expectations color the effects here as in other potentially pleasurable things. One study found that the word "chocolate cake" prompted the response "guilt" in the USA, but "celebration" in France. However, some good effects of alcohol are real.

One randomized, placebo-controlled, double-blind experiment showed that an alcohol dose of 8 g promoted memorizing words related to happiness without any change in general memorizing ability (Warburton 1999). Another double-blind experiment showed that during a six-hour social interaction togetherness was increased by alcohol (Smith et al. 1992). Randomized experiments show that alcohol has good effects. Similar effects can, of course, be produced by friendly company, success in sports, reading a stimulating book, watching a good play and many other things.

Lacking blood alcohol tests, our ancestors relied on human experience in the spirit of know thyself. For example, although the Stoics were not extremely keen on the worldly pleasures, Lucius Annaeus Seneca the Younger (4 BC~ 65 AD) made a distinction between good and bad intoxication (Seneca

71

1964).

> *At times we ought to reach even the point of intoxication, not drowning ourselves in drink, yet succumbing to it; for it washes away troubles, and stirs the mind from its very depths and heals its sorrow just as it does certain ills of the body; and the inventor of wine is not called the Releaser [Liber, Bacchus] on account of the license it gives to the tongue, but because it frees the mind from bondage to cares and emancipates it and gives it new life and makes it bolder in all that it attempts. But, as in freedom, so in wine there is a wholesome moderation... Yet we ought not to do this often, for fear that the mind may contract an evil habit; nevertheless there are times when it must be drawn into rejoicing and freedom, and gloomy sobriety must be banished for a while.*

We could follow his wisdom and draw the line of moderation between drinkers who feel good and behave amiably and those who do not.

7 Not only a poison

It is all in the dosing and time

The temperance people like to stress that alcohol is a poison. True, but only partly true. Many substances are poisons in large amounts but necessary or good in smaller amounts. Water can be poisonous in large amounts. Overdose of a medical drug may kill, while a therapeutic dose heals or alleviates symptoms. It is always a question of dose and time. Some say that alcohol is a poison that kills slowly. I like to respond that fortunately most people are in no hurry.

The temperance people also say if alcohol were discovered now it would be outlawed, so dangerous it is. Sorry folks, then you should also proscribe evolution. It brought about bacteria that need alcohol for their energy. These bacteria can consume approximately 20 % of the energy value of alcohol before it enters the blood stream (Suter et al. 1994). The energy value of alcohol for human beings is therefore lower than the 7 kcal that the dieting books say and what your car gets if it runs on alcohol.

Some bacteria need sugar and produce alcohol from it. In beer and wine-making, this is called fermentation. It happens elsewhere, too. The temperance zealots should outlaw bread made with the help of yeast, yogurt, sourmilk and other stuff containing tiny amounts of alcohol, such as Coca-Cola and

73

"alcohol-free", aka "non-alcoholic", beer. The latter contains usually less than 0.5 % alcohol. We carry in our intestines bacteria that eat sugar and produce alcohol, approximately 3 g daily in the average human being. Other animals do this as well. Stop these walking breweries now! Not possible. Fermentation by bacteria is a part of life. Please, dear advocates of abstinence, remember that if we did not now have alcohol, it should be discovered at once. Alcohol is a good disinfectant, solvent and renewable source of energy, in addition to being good for our health.

74

III

THE DRINKS – HEALTH AND GOOD TASTE

By now we have reviewed the quantity, rhythm and intensity of alcohol intake. To complete the view, let us consider how various kinds of drinks can serve our health, charm our taste and bring about pleasure. Water, tea, coffee, wine, beer and liquor are on. Our taste may be subjective but the knowledge on it is objective. Enjoy your drinking and pass the good practice on to your children!

8 Water - The essence of life

No man is a camel

Living bodies are a mixture of water and other molecules. Water is essential to all life. We need to drink water often. Camels can drink 100 - 200 quarts at a time and then roam weeks, sometimes a month without a refill. All other mammals need water more frequently.

About 50 - 75 % of our body weight is water. An average adult needs approximately 2.5 quarts (or liters) of water daily. Drinking must provide about 1.5 quarts, and the rest comes from food and body metabolism. Old people need to drink daily slightly more than working-age adults because the kidneys concentrate urine less efficiently.

Daily requirement of water depends on environmental temperature and sweating. The body loses more water in higher temperatures, heavy work and long exercise. In these cases, it is good to drink a little water even before you feel thirst. Sports drinks do not normally bring about any extra benefit. Usually about a pint of water (half a liter) per hour is fine, for old people about half a pint. The safe maximum for healthy adults sweating profusely is about 1 - 1.5 quarts per hour. The first warning sign of serious water depletion is the strong yellow color of urine. Colorless urine indicates an overdose of water. Overdosing may lead to water poisoning. Blood becomes too diluted. This can cause brain edema, headache, sleepiness, confusion and muscle cramps, followed in the worst cases by seizures, loss of consciousness and death.

The taste of good water

Purified, distilled water has no color, odor or taste. In fact, no one likes it. Surprisingly, when alcoholic beverages are hard to get or totally lacking, the sales of water distilling apparatuses go up. The devices have other uses, it seems.

Good water contains some oxygen and trace elements. It is not too acidic or alkaline. The taste is refreshing. Cold tap water is the best regular drink, if the quality of communal water is good. Lack of oxygen may make water taste flat. You can increase the oxygen content by stirring. The quality of drinking water can vary much between communities, depending on trace element content and pH.

Trace elements come from soil to ground water. Some trace elements are necessary for life and they improve the taste as well. Too much of trace elements, and the water may taste too salty, bitter, moldy or alkaline. Too much of calcium can make boiled vegetables unpleasantly tough and leave white stains. Water containing a high level of calcium and magnesium is called hard. Soft water is preferable in households.

The amount of free hydrogen ions in water is indicated by the pH score. The score is the inverse logarithm of the ion amount, just for reasons of convenience. The scale is from 0 to

14. When pH is below 7 the solution is acidic and above 7 alkaline. The pH of good drinking water is between 6.5 - 8.6. Tap water is usually slightly alkaline. This keeps the color of boiled vegetables brighter. Too alkaline water will make vegetables mushy, increase the loss of vitamins and make the taste soapy. Alkalinity can be reduced by a few drops of vinegar acid or lemon juice, or some other acidic liquid. If water is too acidic, a pinch of baking soda to a gallon (or 4 - 5 liters) of water may suffice to correct it.

Many soft drinks, wine and beer are acidic. Acids make the drinks fresh but can harm dental enamel. The lower the pH, the higher the risk. *Table 4*, in the chapter on gout, shows the approximate pH values in various drinks. Sugar is another enemy of the enamel. It is a good idea to either abstain from acidic and sweet drinks completely or drink them only during meals.

Tasting and smelling water tells much about its quality. Experienced human tasters are the ultimate arbiters of quality, except for the presence of bacteria and viruses. If bacterial contamination is suspected water has to be boiled. Bacteria will not multiply if you store drinking water at the temperature of 34 - 39 °F (1 - 4 °C).

9 Wine, beer and liquor - The milk of adults

Not only water and alcohol.

The best nutrient for infants is mother's milk, but for adults milk is white poison. Blood vessels will become hard and narrow, the heart will suffer. The small amount of alcohol in your favorite beverage, be it beer, wine, liquor or something else, will keep the vessels healthy longer. In addition, several of these beverages contain also trace elements, vitamins, carbohydrates, proteins and phenolic substances that may have beneficial effects.

Polyphenols are a group of complex alcohol molecules and at least 500 are known. They protect plants from insects and give color. Good sources include apples, onions, celery *(Apium graveolens var. dulce)*, cabbage family, cranberry, black tea and dark chocolate. One study found that the one-third of people with highest polyphenol intake from food had 20 % (95 % CI 0.69 - 0.93) lower cardiovascular mortality than the one-third with lowest intake (Huxley and Neil 2003).

Wine contains a long list of different polyphenols, and their effects are many (Rodrigo et al. 2011). The polyphenol content in red wine is on average higher than in white wine because in red wine fermentation the juice remains in contact with grape skins longer. Beer and some liquors have small amounts of polyphenols. Not all polyphenols are absorbed

81

from the gut to blood and thus do not have internal (systemic) effects. The remaining part may influence the gut bacteria in several, mostly yet unknown, ways. Some of these may be beneficial.

Many follow-up studies on human population groups have found that preference of wine or beer is related to better health and lower mortality than other preferences, even when the long-term average alcohol intake has been controlled for (Grønbæk et al. 1995; Klatsky and Armstrong 1989; Poikolainen and Vartiainen 1999; Strandberg et al. 2007; Ruidavets et al. 2010). But results favoring beer and liquor drinkers have also been found (Rimm et al. 1996).

It seems to be very difficult to identify the pure effect of wine polyphenols on health in epidemiological studies. The intake of polyphenols from alcoholic beverages is small compared with that from food. Most drinkers do not stick to only one beverage type or brand of drink. The effects of alcohol, drinking rhythm and speed of drinking confound comparisons. Drinkers preferring some particular drink may differ in some other ways, too. One study found that wine drinkers had less coronary heart disease risk factors than drinkers preferring other beverages (Wannamethee and Shaper 1999). Another study found that wine drinkers, compared with others, bought more food considered healthy, such as fish, fruit, vegetables and olive oil (Tjønneland et al. 1999). The epidemiological studies on the incidence of disease and death have not provided any clear answers, although they suggest that red wine might have more benefits than other drinks.

Wine, beer and liquor can make interesting drinks when blended with water. Try any natural wine or beer you like, add a liberal amount of water. Find out the proportions of the blend you like best. Compare the straight beverage and different diluted blends. You might find that a good deal of the original taste is preserved in the blends. Whisky tasters often make fifty-fifty blends when judging the quality. The Hungarians have a great tradition of drinking water-wine mixtures of various strengths, just like the ancient Greeks did.

10 Coffee, tea and energy drinks - The soft stimulants

Light stimulation is good rather than bad for most.

Both coffee and tea contain polyphenols and caffeine. Caffeine stimulates, increases energy production in muscles and speeds up reactions. Overdose may cause anxiety, nervousness, headache, difficulty to fall asleep, high heart rate and a small temporary increase in blood pressure. The maximum effect of one dose will take place from 15 minutes to two hours after drinking. About 100 mg of caffeine is enough to strengthen the effect of painkiller medicines. No one should take more than 1000 mg of caffeine daily. Pregnant women should not exceed 300 mg daily. This, or even smaller doses, may cause restlessness and other side effects in people especially susceptible to the effects of caffeine.

The amount of caffeine varies in coffee, depending on the type of beans, roasting, brewing method and the size of the cup. Roughly, the amount of caffeine in a regular cup (whatever it might be) is for

- ordinary coffee   65 - 175 mg
- espresso   80 - 115 mg
- tea   50 mg
- cola drink   40 - 50 mg

- cocoa   15 mg.

There is no standard cup size. An American measuring cup contains 237 ml, a metric one 250 ml. An ordinary European coffee cup might be 150 ml and a tea cup 250 ml. A typical espresso cup size is 60 ml. In China, a small 25 ml teacup is not uncommon but 150 - 200 ml cups are also popular. Most adults can drink 3 - 4 cups of coffee or tea without any harmful effects.

Coffee contains fats. Of these, cafestol and kahweol enter the blood stream and add to the harms from cholesterol except when coffee is made by letting it drip through a filter (Bonita et al. 1997). One randomized study found that after drinking strong unfiltered coffee 5- 6 cups daily for six months, the bad low-density lipoprotein (LDL) cholesterol level increased by 9 - 14 %. No changes were observed in the comparison group drinking filtered coffee (56). Such a high exposure to unfiltered coffee may be exceptionally infrequent. At customary intake levels, coffee has been found not to increase the risk of coronary heart disease (Kleemola et al. 2000).

Coffee may decrease the risk of adult-type diabetes, Parkinson's disease, liver cirrhosis and liver cell cancer (Higdon and Frei 2006). This may be due to either polyphenols or some yet unknown substances. The taste of coffee and tea is mostly due to the polyphenol content although the quality of water also plays a role. A daily cup of cocoa may slightly decrease blood pressure (2 - 3 mmHg). Polyphenols might also be responsible for this effect (Ried et al. 2012). Drinking tea

85

has been found to decrease the risk of coronary heart disease, stroke, Parkinson's disease, cancers of the lung, breast and prostate gland as well as all-cause mortality among men but not among women (Qui et al. 2012). Do not drink your coffee or tea too hot. High temperature may increase the risk of cancers of the upper digestive tract. The temperature should be less than 122 °F (50° C). Stir the beverage or add cold water if you are in a hurry and cannot wait.

Concoctions called energy drinks have recently become popular. Marketing promises stamina, muscle power and alertness. All these drinks contain a modest amount of caffeine, often equaling one cup of coffee. Other constituents vary. There might be taurine, dimethylamylamine, creatine, β-alanine, sugar, vitamins or some phosphates. Most acute effects seem to be due to caffeine. In one study caffeine made reactions faster but taurine tended to attenuate this effect (Peacock et al. 2013). Joint intake of energy drinks and alcohol has become popular among some youth circles. Energy drinks may increase the acute stimulating effect of alcohol or lessen the subsequent sedation. Health risks are poorly known but adverse effects on the heart, blood pressure and behavior are possible if intake is high. Research on the effects of energy drinks is sparse. Most studies are small and pertain to acute effects only. Long-term effects remain unknown.

11 What is good taste

Learn to enjoy more.

Evolution has provided us with the ability to enjoy food and drink. Otherwise we could not survive long. People who have lost their faculty of taste do not always eat and drink enough. Old people often have to be fed. Let us now see how taste functions and what is understood by good taste.

From stimuli to perception

When a taste-triggering chemical substance meets the receptor in a sensory nerve ending, transmission of a nerve impulse begins. The tongue and the inside wall of the mouth have on average 600,000 receptors for the basic tastes and touch. The former include sweet, sour, salty, bitter and umami (savory taste). Receptors are found all over in the mouth, not at specific sites in the tongue. The touch receptors respond also to temperature, pain and astringent (desiccating) stimuli. Astringent feeling differs from bitter. You can feel a strong drying sensation, for example, when eating raw banana or drinking strong black tea or young red wine. It is born when tannins or other polyphenols make the proteins in saliva combine into larger molecules. The touch sensation can also be soft or crisp.

87

We talk about basic tastes because the total taste sensation includes also touch and smell. The overall phenomenon is called flavor by some professionals. In the nose, about six million olfactory receptors respond to smell chemicals. Odors seem different depending on whether the chemicals enter the nose directly or behind through the back of the mouth. On average, we humans can identify a few hundred different odors. One perfume tester is said to identify seven hundred. Smell receptors are crucial in tasting. You will notice this clearly when you catch a flu. Hardly anything is sensed except perhaps sourness. Even in normal conditions, the taste sense easily becomes tired. Receptors die and new are born every few days. The number of receptors and taste sensitivity decline with age.

Perceived taste in our consciousness is the end result of many nerve pathways. There is no one-to-one relationship. The perception of taste is a strongly edited version, colored and selected by our mind. Seeing and hearing may also influence the final taste perception.

There are two components in perception - intensity and quality. Quality is either pleasant, indifferent or unpleasant. Professionals call this hedonic valence. Depending on whether the valence is positive or negative, we may call the sensation a perfume, scent or stink. Some say that depending on the preconditions one certain scent can be interpreted either as Parmesan cheese or vomit. Much depends on the intensity of the sensation. Wines from the grape Sauvignon blanc may

88

charm because of a cat pee smell and old Pinot Noir because of a certain whiff of *merde de cheval,* that is horse manure, pardon my French.

Tasting performance

There is a wide range between individuals in tasting performance. To identify a certain taste by name, stronger stimuli are needed than only to detect the presence of some taste. Detection threshold differences can vary 1000-fold between individuals. Some people are called supertasters only because they perceive a certain chemical (phenylthiocarbimide) bitter while others do not. Supertasters are also especially sensitive to sweetness and sourness. Supertasters avoid smoking, alcoholic beverages and foods that taste bitter. They are also choosy in what they eat. However, they are not generally superior to other tasters. Approximately 25 - 30 % of the population are supertasters. The feature seems to be genetic. While tasting performance is partly due to genes, also experience and practice play a role.

Our preferences for what we like to drink and eat differ a lot. This is normal. Opinions differ but everybody is right in what he or she likes best. Even food critics as well as wine and beer experts have their differences in quality and ratings. Just compare what two international gurus say about the same product. It has been said that even more differences might be revealed if our vocabulary to describe tastes were not so

89

limited (Goode 2008).

Descriptions and quality ratings

We describe taste by analogy, searching for associations between the drink under study and other substances. Do the taste and odor resemble that of certain fruits, berries, flowers, hays, trees, spices or other biological or artificial substances? Similarities can sometimes be due to a certain chemical substance but are often a result of several substances, some unknown, and the perception can be a result of the mutual interaction between several factors. Odors from nature can consist of hundreds of chemicals. The odor of rancid butter is not exactly the same as white wine after malolactic fermentation despite both containing diacetyl. The odor of green pepper differs from red wine from Cabernet sauvignon grapes in spite of the presence of 2-metoxy-3-isobutylpyrazine in both. For some wine and beer odors we do not find any comparison from nature. The odors are simply unique (Amerine and Roessler 1976).

Associative comparisons may remain pale. Judgments are enriched by value-laden words to indicate the hedonic valence. The interpretative processes in the mind influence the final description. The end result much depends on what the judge thinks, believes or suspects. Frédéric Brochet (1999) has shown that beliefs on the type, price and color of wine play a major role. White wine, made red by artificial color, was described by words typical of red wine (Brochet and Dubourdieu 2001, Morrot et al. 2001). Sensory evaluation is sensitive to biases. The most reliable results are reached when the jury members work alone in their silent, odorless cubicles, without any prior knowledge. Blinding or blue or black glasses can be used to camouflage the color of the drink.

Overall quality is often expressed in numeral ratings (Peynaud 1987). This is not totally unbiased. Different types of beverages cannot be compared without difficulty. The range of rating scale scores varies. The following scales are commonly used

- one to five (often stars)
- 0 - 20
- 10 - 20
- 0 - 100
- 50 - 100.

The scales are typically constructed by adding scores given to color, odor, taste and overall impression together. One scale may give more weight to odor, another to taste. One thing is common to all scales. The higher the rating, the better the drink sells. For some people, a 90-point wine seems to taste much better than an 89-point one.

Dimensions of taste

Are there general properties that describe excellence in taste

91

experience? There is no definite theory of taste esthetics. However, Peter Klosse (2004) has constructed one model. He suggests that there are three dimensions in wine flavor:

- Flavor richness - its components include basic tastes, odors and mouth feel

- Contracting sensation - its components include acids, polyphenols and salt

- Coating sensation - its components include sugars, fats, fruit flavors, alcohol and glycerol

On the basis of the above, Klosse has constructed a 2 x 2 x 2 flavor cube that divides wines into eight types. For example, wines with low coating but with high richness and contracting sensation can be described as spicy, hot and explosive. Low contracting but high coating and rich wines are filling, full and ripe in flavor. When there is an abundance of all three components the wine is complex and balanced.

Similar components can be found in beer. Contracting elements include acids, bitter aromas from hops, polyphenols, and fruity banana and apple aromas. Alcohol, sugar, and buttery diacetyl give coating sensations. Roasted malt delivers caramel, chocolate and smoke aromas. Many aroma-producing chemicals have been identified (Briggs et al. 2004). Mouth feel is much influenced by the amount of carbon dioxide.

Richness often wins nowadays over complexity and

balance in evaluations in the press. "More is better" dominates the thinking of many a critic. Let us not forget that harmony is one feature of good-tasting beverage. David Hume (1711 ~ 1776) pointed this out when he wrote that *"A good palate is not tried by strong flavors, but by a mixture of small ingredients, where we are still sensible of each part, notwithstanding its minuteness and its confusion with the rest."* (Hume, *Essays, moral, political, and literary.* I.XXIII.18.).

93

12 Should teenagers be allowed to taste alcoholic beverages - Consider carefully

Parental skills are called for.

Children notice what happens when parents drink. Parents are responsible for setting an example and advising their children. A good guide is the *Addiction-proof your Child* by Stanton Peele (2007). One question needs more consideration. Should teenagers be allowed to taste alcoholic beverages? I feel that it is a good thing to do if there is sufficient mutual trust and harmony in the family, and if the amount is a few small sips, diluted in water, if considered appropriate.

A common fallacy is that the earlier a teenager tastes alcoholic beverages, the higher the risk of alcoholism. This derives from studies that have asked about the onset of drinking without making a distinction between tasting and intoxication. Better studies have shown that it is the intoxicating drinking, not tasting, that increases risk (Warner and White 2003; Rossow and Kuntsche 2013; Morean eat al. 2012). While this is true, earlier antecedents of drunkenness can be found, emerging before any exposure to alcohol. The risk of alcoholism is increased by aggression, difficult temperament, conduct problems, hyperactivity and low intelligence as well as parental alcoholism and child-rearing that is punishing, unjust, inconsistent or indifferent (Rossow and Kuntsche 2013; Poikolainen 2002; White et al. 2011). The devil resides in us, not in the bottle.

Is alcohol more dangerous to children and teenagers than to adults? No one knows. Ethical reasons forbid experiments on the young ones. As noted above, the young who drink heavily differ from other young people already before the onset of drinking. It is probably impossible to control for all these confounding factors. We could hardly find enough young people for comparison who drink heavily but lack all other possible risk factors. Studies of intoxicated teenagers in hospital treatment suggest that at this age people are more resistant to the acute overdose effects than when older. Rat experiments have been interpreted to support the opposite view. At least one of these studies has been found to jump to conclusions in opposition to its results (Uhl 2009). The lesson from this is that never believe the abstract of a scientific study unless you are convinced that the methods and results agree with the former. And if you still suspect the results, look whether other studies agree, prove otherwise or are inconclusive. There is a lot of intention-to-cheat analysis around.

Most studies support the view that alcohol education in schools is useless. Advice should be given earlier at home before puberty. I think that this works well if relations between children and parents are reasonably good. Protect your children from good-for-nothing friends and school temperance education.

I remember well one evening long ago when my wife

95

and I opened a bottle of red wine to have with our meal. Both our children become very anxious. They had not seen anything like this before. However, they soon relaxed when all went peacefully without brouhaha in contrast to what they had recently been taught at school. When the children became adults, they could recall the happy family get-togethers as in an old Burgundian song from the 17th century.

> *Ah! Que nos pères étaient heureux*
> *Quand ils étaient à table.*
> *Le vin coulait au milieu d'eux*
> *Ça leur était fort agréable.*
> Oh! How happy were our parents
> Around the family dinner table.
> Connected by wine like currents
> this being for them most enjoyable.[8]

---

[8] My translation from the original. Source: Berthat H. *Vingt chansons du vin de Bourgogne*. Dijon: Èditions Latitudes-L'Harmattan, 1995.

96

IV
PROTECT YOURSELF

98

Not long ago, bad things happened to a man who thought that honesty is the best policy. When asked about his drinking by his M.D., he said that he had six beers daily, although only on weekends. Some months later, a letter informed the 44-year old man that his driver's license had been suspended because of his alcohol problem. He had driven 22 years without an accident and always sober. He thought that drinking beer in his own home was his business alone. The court thought otherwise. They required that this honest man spend three months in substance abuse treatment, paid fully by himself, as a condition for license renewal. This took place in Pennsylvania.[9] Could this somehow happen to you?

Do not readily reveal your alcohol intake to other people. Beware of *AUDIT* and other brief questionnaires, for such screening instruments exaggerate the risks of drinking. As a consequence, you may be falsely labeled as a risk drinker or an alcoholic. See Part VI for what sort of people alcoholics really are. Also watch out for so-called brief advice to reduce alcohol intake, frequently offered in primary and occupational health care. It exposes you to the risk of labeling and the practice of less-than-perfect drinking. Keep in mind ways to defend yourself.

Do not take seriously the so-called 'liver enzyme' values as an indicator of excessive alcohol intake. The most common of these blood tests is Gamma-glutamyltransferase (GGT). Its

---

[9] On http://www.post-gazette.com/pg/04196/346128.stm. [Accessed Aug 14, 2004]. The page no longer exists.

99

values correlate poorly with alcohol intake (Poikolainen et al. 1985). Values moderately above the upper normal reference limit do not clearly point to any specific health problem. Elevated values may be due to tobacco smoking, obesity, intake of some common drugs or several diseases (Kunutsor 2016). If values are very high it is best to consult with your doctor. Other common 'liver enzymes' that correlate poorly with alcohol intake are alanine transaminase (ALT), aspartate transaminase (AST). All these are much more unreliable indicators of alcohol intake than self-reports.

Part I dealt with the major effects of alcohol intake on health to help you decide the quantity and rhythm of drinking you consider best. To hold your intake at this level it is wise to monitor your drinking and even keep a log. Tips on how to do this follow. You can apply either an exact method or more approximate one. Part V reviews the risks of alcohol intake for several diseases, accidents and violence. Part VI covers the causes and cures of alcoholism. Finally, Part VII points out that mistaken alcohol policy overlooks the main problem and undermines the life of moderate drinkers.

13 Avoid AUDIT and brief advice in health care

Screening for alcohol problems can jeopardize your rights.

As noted earlier, many recommended drinking levels have been published. The need arose when someone thought that it would be a good idea to have family doctors advise their patients to cut down on alcohol intake. I suspect that the model was copied from anti-smoking advice. "Stop smoking" is a simple and relevant message, while "stop drinking" would not have worked. Thus the need was felt to find out how much drinking is too much, how to identify patients exceeding the limit and how to push them below it. The trade name for the push is brief advice to reduce alcohol intake. It aims to give advice in primary and occupational health care.

It is believed that the primary care physician has more influence over patient behavior than do other advisers. Other unsubstantiated assumptions are as follows: (i) harmful alcohol use becomes progressively worse and harder to treat year by year, being totally or almost impossible to treat when the final stage of alcohol dependence has been reached, and (ii) the earlier advice is given, the better the results. Intuitively there seems to be some logic in this train of thought. However, there is no solid evidence for better results due to earlier rather than later interventions. On the contrary, research has shown that the track of alcohol intake over the years varies much between individuals. Progressive increase is not commonly observed. Typically, young single adults are most keen on partying and drinking to excess. Most of them moderate their alcohol intake later without any kind of treatment because of work and marital commitments. Risky drinking is not a condition where the idea "the earlier, the better" works well. It works only with diseases that have a silent (unsymptomatic) early stage. Nevertheless, a medical doctor who is used to the reflex hammer sees only tendon reflexes as the problem.

Drinking problems are screened, not discovered by *AUDIT*

Several short questionnaires have been developed, to distinguish between potential problem drinkers and other persons. The most popular of these is the *Alcohol Use Disorders Identification Test*, abbreviated to *AUDIT*. It aims to screen cases with hazardous or harmful drinking, not alcoholics (Saunders et al. 1993). The good news is that is has spread all over the world as widely as influenza. The bad news is that it is a spectacular failure. It does not meet the requirements of a good test for screening.

A proper screening test aims to detect a subclinical disease, something that has not yet caused any symptoms. Alcohol problems have no unsymptomatic prodromal stage.

While screening can be useful for the early detection of diseases, say cancer, that later produce symptoms, a good deal of young problem drinkers mature out of their harmful drinking patterns all by themselves. Not so with cancer patients.

Table 3. AUDIT-C questions and scoring

How often do you have a drink containing alcohol?

never = 0	once a month or less often = 1	2-4 times a month = 2	2-3 times a week = 3	4 times a week or more often = 4

How many drinks containing alcohol do you have on a typical day when you are drinking?

1-2 drinks = 0	3-4 drinks = 1	5-6 drinks = 2	7-9 drinks = 3	10+ drinks = 4

How often have you had six or more drinks on one occasion?

never = 0	once a month or less often = 1	once a month = 2	once a week = 3	daily or almost daily = 4

When *AUDIT* was developed, it was validated against a mixed bag of outcomes. The "disease" to be screened included persons who in their own view thought that they drank abnormally, had a drinking problem, drank daily more than 60 g of alcohol, or at least once a week 120 g or more, were

103

repeatedly intoxicated or had at least one of the "symptoms" of alcohol dependence. This kind of trap will catch a fairly large share of population. The problem is that then you should separate the edible fish from the rest, that is the true positives needing advice from the false positives. After all, *AUDIT* was intended to be a screening test.

Many family doctors are in a great hurry and would prefer something quicker than *AUDIT*. Thus *AUDIT-C* was born. It is simply the first three questions of *AUDIT*. These pertain to alcohol intake (*Table 3*) and are too rough to yield any useful estimate of actual consumption. The parent *AUDIT* contains, in addition, three questions on harmful consequences and four on behaviors related to alcohol dependence.

Brief advice wastes resources and may be hazardous to health

How well do *AUDIT* and *AUDIT-C* perform as screening instruments in primary health care? Let us assume that there are 10,000 patients in a family practice, of which 500 problem drinkers and 500 are alcoholics. On the condition of the original study of *AUDIT*, sensitivity is 80 % and specificity 98 % when the screening cutpoint is 10. This was based on combined results from six countries (Saunders et al. 1993). In this case, *AUDIT* detects as screening positives 800 cases with either problem drinking or alcoholism and in addition 180 persons who are false positives. Brief advice for one person requires two visits, both probably lasting for 10 - 15 minutes. To motivate one alcoholic into substance abuse treatment calls for one visit at least. Under these assumptions, 14.7 % of all available patient visits are taken up by dealing with alcohol issues (1.5 times 980 visits). If the performance of *AUDIT* follows the findings of an Italian study, then the alcohol visits consume 26 % of all available visits to the family doctor (Piccinelli et al. 1997). If the practice applies *AUDIT-C* and its screening cutpoint 3 to save time, 3 740 positive cases would be detected according to screening performance (Gordon et al. 2001). Of these, 3 075 would meet the cutpoint of 4 and thus be false or true positives for alcohol dependence (Dawson et al. 2012). Allocating again one visit per one suspected case of alcohol dependence and two for the other positives, 44 % of all doctor visits are needed to process this group.

One study has suggested that brief advice works well also for alcoholics. In this case, all screening positives should be given two visits. That would take up 75 % of all visits. All the above was based on the assumption that 10 % of the population has an alcohol problem. If the actual percentage is 15 %, the share of the screened group would be 81 % of all visits. The percentage may soon be even higher. The brand new American diagnostic system DSM-5 combines problem drinking and alcohol dependence into a diagnosis called alcohol use disorder. This is expected to classify more people into the group that should understand that they need treatment.

105

The catch seems to be 11- 18 % of the adult population in the USA. Other factors expanding the number of customers are, first, that *AUDIT-C* is often taken to show that the problem has been diagnosed, not that the screening results reveal that there might be a problem. Secondly, there seems to be a tendency to decrease the cutpoints. What benefits would brief advice to this broadening group bring about?

The most recent meta-analysis included 34 studies and showed that participants who received brief intervention consumed only 3 g/day less alcohol than minimal or no intervention participants after one year according to the self-reports (Kaner al. 2018). There was no difference in the gamma-glutamyltransferase levels, a test that correlates with alcohol intake. The mean alcohol intake level at the beginning of the trials was 37 g/day. In an earlier meta-analysis, comprising 23 randomzed studies, mean alcohol intake at the beginning of the trials was 35 g/day. In all these studies, the average alcohol intake in the advice groups before brief advice visits remained lower than the largest available meta-analysis risk level estimate of 50 - 75 g/day. Only in two studies did this intake exceed 45 g/day. On average, advice decreased intake to the level of 32 - 36 g/day (Jonas et al. 2012). In some cases, following advice would decrease intake to levels less than the optimal intake.

The randomized studies show some trivial positive effect for brief interventions. These studies are carried out in ideal conditions by enthusiastic staff. However, the everyday practice is different. An observational study in the USA found that brief intervention based on AUDIT-C scores was not effective in real-world conditions (Williams et al. 2014).

The main task in primary health care is to focus on the fundamental complaint of the patient. If the visit starts with something else the patient will be confused and disappointed. In Britain, physicians have strongly criticized such efforts to change the primary focus (Public health in England: from nudge to nag. *Lancet* 2012). The correct place for brief advice is not in primary health care. Other places, such as the internet, serve better. Brief advice wastes the scarce resources of primary health care and may in some cases be hazardous to health.

How should I respond?

The egregious misuse of *AUDIT* and other screening instruments poses a risk. You may be labeled a risk drinker, problem drinker, alcohol dependent or something similar. Some health professionals take moralistic stands and blame patients who have other moral values and preferences than they themselves do. Negative attitude might be reflected on how you are being treated. Be forthcoming only if you can trust your doctor and his or her ability to respect confidentiality. Otherwise, do not reveal or consider under-reporting your intake if you feel that this is the best way. In the ideal world, patients and doctors should follow the outspoken norms in their encounters. Patients should answer honestly to all questions

107

and do their best to co-operate in treatment. Doctors should observe strict confidentiality and do their best to treat the patient. Alas, actual situations often differ from this ideal. In London, more than seven in 10 primary care doctors think that their patients under-report their alcohol intake.[10]

Ignore negative reactions. Remember that some health professionals may have misunderstood what is the difference between risk and causation, as explained earlier. And that they often rely on what the abstracts of research papers claim, without having the time to critically assess the complete literature base. Record your alcohol intake, keep it under your hat and compare your intake with your own health. Next, see how you can record what you drink.

---

[10] http://www.aim-digest.com/digest/pdigest/current/Sep18diges t.pdf

14 Count and record your own alcohol intake

Self-monitoring keeps you in control.

If you want exact figures on how much alcohol enters your body start a process of observation, calculation and record-keeping. The task is to turn raw data into grams of alcohol per day. Then it can easily be compared with estimates of risk presented in Part I. Record the volume of your drinks, the alcohol content (as shown on the bottle label) and apply the formula below:

Alcohol in grams = 0.079 times (volume of the beverage imbibed, in centiliters) times (alcohol content of the beverage, in percent of volume).

If you favor a limited number of beverages and your glass size does not vary you will soon remember how many grams your drinks contain. If you prefer easier, less accurate methods, there are at least three possibilities.

1. A rough rule of thumb: One centiliter of wine contains one gram of alcohol, one centiliter of beer one-third of a gram, and one centiliter of liquor three grams.
2. The standard drink method: Find out what is the alcohol content of a standard drink in your country. In England one unit contains approximately 8 g, in Australia 10 g, in the USA 12 g (some accept 14 g), in Canada 13.6 g

109

and in Japan 20 g. Bars and restaurants usually serve standard measures of alcoholic beverages. Record the number of standard drinks you have had and calculate the multiple of drinks and its alcohol content in grams.

3. Internet: Let some calculator on the internet do the job for you. Some of them are rather sophisticated, allowing you to choose the type and brand of the beverage. You only have to remember to make notes on the beverage volumes and brands consumed.

110

V

RISKS, HIGH AND LOW

112

Imagine that you get lost on a hiking trip in a wild forest, and you have to decide how to find your way out. There seem to be three possibilities for this. You may camp on a small river you have found and wait for rescue, or there is a canoe and you can paddle downriver. Or, you might hike in a direction where you think there is a road. You must consider carefully the likelihood of success and risk in each of these options. Which option you take depends on the probability of various outcomes and the subjective value you attach to it, if you rely on logical reasoning, like economists do. Think, do you prefer hiking and eating wild berries and are not scared of bears, or prefer being lazy and fishing and assume someone comes to the rescue, or opt for paddling and hope you face no rapids. Having arrived at these hunches, you count the product of the probabilities and values to yield utilities and choose the one with the highest score. It is the best option for you according to the rules of rational decision-making.

In the same vein, you might consider the risk of any behavior and practice. What good and what bad consequences you can expect, how likely are they and what are the subjective values of these consequences for you. For example, are there factors increasing the risk of a particular disease, how much does a certain level of these factors increase the risk, and how would you feel if you became ill. Few people employ these rational gymnastics that economists of the neoclassic school suppose we do all the time. The calculations are not simple ones, you seldom have enough accurate information and

113

probabilities are necessarily based on past experience and intuition. The future might be different. Despite these obstacles, it is useful to find out what is known, consider the preferences and risks and sleep on it. Often this lets the intuitive problem-solving system in your subconscious work out a reasonable solution.

Part I dealt with the general health effects of alcohol intake and with major diseases related to the decreased risk of ill-health. It is now time to look at main negative outcomes of alcohol intake. Heavy drinking is one major cause of liver cirrhosis, some cancers, gout, road accidents, violence and aggression as well as harmful effects to the newborn due to drinking during pregnancy. But there are other causes than alcohol, too. And there are ways to decrease the risk of these harms. Moreover, some low levels of drinking are materially harmless.

15 The many causes of liver cirrhosis

Liver disease has many risk factors, including a protective one.
.

The liver is the powerhouse of the body. It breaks down complex food molecules, assembles the components into new molecules that the body needs, and it eliminates poisons. Cirrhosis is a process that renders some production lines ineffective and finally defunct. More and more liver cells fail to do their job. During the early stage, failures are not yet large and there are no symptoms. The diagnosis is difficult. Many a cirrhosis case is found only in autopsy. Cirrhosis may be suspected only when symptoms, such as weight loss, lack of appetite, general weakness, yellow skin or blood in vomit are present. The best evidence of cirrhosis is obtained by taking a sample of liver tissue with a needle (biopsy). It is not painless, not fully safe and not absolutely sure to harvest cirrhotic tissue from the liver. But it is the strongest evidence we have. After cirrhosis has been found it is imperative to abstain from alcohol. Abstinence will increase survival considerably. Death is often due to loss of blood from the veins in the esophagus or liver cancer.

At present, everyone knows that alcohol is a major cause of liver cirrhosis. Earlier, until the 1980's, the common medical view was that the cause must be something else. Findings showing fairly high correlations between alcohol consumption

115

and liver cirrhosis mortality, both between countries and over consecutive years in one country, were thought to be just statistical correlations, not a cause. There were several reasons. Some studies found no correlation and some others negative correlations (de Lint 1981; Chick 1993). High alcohol doses did not bring about cirrhosis in the rat or in the mouse. Nutritional deficiencies were suspected since malnourished humans had cirrhosis more often than those with an adequate diet.

The pivotal act was to study baboons. Charles Lieber (1931 ~ 2009) and his team were able to produce the findings necessary to turn the heads of the medical community. No cirrhosis was observed during oral administration of alcohol and solid food. Only when alcohol and liquid nutrients (half of the energy from both sources) were administered into the vein, five baboons out of 15 developed hepatitis and another five cirrhosis (Lieber et al. 1975). I'd like to know whether the lack of fiber in the liquid diet had some influence on the result. Fiber decreases the risk of cancers in the gut. Alcoholics are no great fans of fresh fruit, vegetables and rye bread, all good sources of fiber.

Later, epidemiological cohort and case-control studies have explored the alcohol-cirrhosis relation in more detail. The results are not consistent. Some studies have found progressively increasing relations, sometimes linear, other times exponential. But two studies have found that there is a ceiling: after an initial increase by augmenting alcohol intake the risk of cirrhosis stopped rising and leveled out (Sørensen 1989; Kamper-Jørgensen et al. 2004). As to cirrhosis mortality, the ceiling was found at the intake level of 60 g/day (Lelbach 1975).

One case-control study suggests that it is not easy to develop cirrhosis. It found that the incidence of cirrhosis was linearly related to the lifetime amount of alcohol divided by body weight (Klatsky and Armstrong 1992). The results suggest that the risk of cirrhosis is 50 % if a man weighing 154 lb (70 kg) drinks daily 180 g of alcohol over 25 years. This would be approximately 16 drinks daily. If drinking continues at this level for 45 years the risk is almost 100 %. The total lifetime amount of 100 % alcohol for our man would be about 3000 kg. On the other hand, the risk seemed to be practically zero if the daily amount were 20 g for 45 years. This agrees with the fact that alcoholic cirrhosis tends to manifest itself in old age.

Women are more prone to develop cirrhosis than men. For them, the risky drinking levels may be something like one half or one third of those for men. However, risk of liver cirrhosis has been found to be approximately 50 % lower among those drinking mainly with meals than those not, lower among wine drinkers than among other drinkers, and lower among those not drinking every day than the rest (Simpson et al. 2019). This seems also relevant for men.

Other risk factors for cirrhosis include viral infections of the liver, such as hepatitis B, C and perhaps E, smoking,

117

obesity, proton-pump inhibitor medication to decrease stomach acidity, malnutrition, some environmental poisons, like aflatoxin, and perhaps genetic factors, and some intestinal bacteria or the toxins produced by them. Lack of enough REC3G lectin to control intestinal bacteria in control may lead in damage in long term. Smoking 20 cigarettes/day has been found to relate to 4-fold risk increase among women in England (Liu et al. 2009). Coffee consumption has been found to decrease the risk of cirrhosis (Klatsky and Armstrong 1992; Corrao et al. 1994).

16 Some cancers are alcohol-related

International Agency for Research on Cancer (IARC) has classified (ethyl-) alcohol into the first and most dangerous class of carcinogenic substances in 2009. To put this in context, note that in this class you will also find soot, wood dust, leather dust, formaldehyde (commonly found in the building material chipboard), chrome and nickel (found in wrist watches), estrogen (used for hormone replacement treatment), and the breast-cancer drug tamoxifen. Large doses of alcohol increase the risk of some cancers, small doses do not. For some cancers, the risk is lower among moderate drinkers than among abstainers.

Alcohol increases the risk of cancer mainly in the upper parts of our food-processing tube spanning from the mouth to the anus. The tube is inside us but outside our veritable inner body. The environment in the tube is totally different, populated by more bacteria than our body has cells. Some of the bacteria produce the energy they need by oxidizing alcohol to acetaldehyde. It is the acetaldehyde that is the villain. Cancer risk depends on how much acetaldehyde is produced and where it is produced. The high risk area is the beginning of the tube, generally called the upper digestive tract, consisting of mouth, pharynx, and esophagus. Acetaldehyde production is increased by smoking and genetic variations that bring about high

119

acetaldehyde concentrations in the blood. These variations are common among some Oriental people. The combined risk of smoking and alcohol is higher than that of either one alone. Risk is also increased by very hot drinks (above 150 °F/65 °C) (Islami et al. 2009).

One meta-analysis found that the overall cancer risk (incidence and mortality) does not differ significantly between abstainers and drinkers with an intake level of 25 g /day. At the level of 50 g /day the respective risk ratios (abstainers = 1) were as follows (men/women).

- mouth and pharynx   2.85
- larynx   1.94
- esophagus   1.98/2.24
- stomach   1.05
- colon and rectum   1.18
- liver   1.51/3.57
- breast   - /1.67
- ovaries, women   1.23
- prostate, men   1.09
- all cancer forms   1.22

No significant risk increase was found for the cancers of small intestine, gallbladder, pancreas, lung, cervix of the uterus, urinary bladder or kidney (Bagnardi et al. 2001). This meta-analysis included studies conducted between the years 1966 - 2000 but not the gigantic *American Cancer Society*

Study (Thun et al.1997). In the latter, at the level of 48 g/ day the risk of upper digestive tract cancers was 2.8-fold among men and 3-fold among women. This agrees well with the above meta-analysis. The *Million Women Study,* a British understatement because the number of women was actually 1.3 million, found that incidence of all cancers was slightly (4 %) higher among abstainers than among women drinking two units (16 g) or less in a week. Risk was increased if intake was seven units (56 g) or more in a week (Allen et al. 2009).

Breast cancer

Breast cancer is the most common female cancer in many countries. It is much feared, but treatment results are rather good. Risk factors include environmental radiation, x-rays, genes, lack of childbirth, hormone replacement therapy, overweight and alcohol intake. There are no strong risk factors. Alcohol intake does not increase the risk much. In the *American Cancer Society Study*, no increase was found for alcohol even at the level of 48 g/ day (Thun et al. 1997). In the cohort of over 85,000 nurses in the USA, the female breast cancer risk was 1.67-fold (95% CI 1.10 - 1.94) among women consuming 30 g or more daily, compared with non-drinkers (Fuchs et al. 1995). In a follow-up study of almost 23,000 women with breast cancer, alcohol intake did not have any influence on the rate of death, neither before nor after the diagnosis. Women who increased their alcohol intake after the diagnosis lived longer than abstainers. Intake was light, the

121

highest group consuming 10 drinks or more a week (Newcomb et al. 2013).

17 Gout - The revenge of affluence

The big toe suddenly becomes hot, red and swollen. This is gout for you. Last night complete with good food and booze, and now there is pain from head to toe. Gout likes to attack the coldest parts of the body, so it searches for the toes. Cold makes urate in the blood precipitate into crystals, bringing about inflammation. Pain is sudden and lasts for several days if not treated. Non-steroidal painkillers ease the pain. But hold your horses if this was your first attack. Some other diseases may produce similar symptoms. To confirm the diagnosis have the synovial fluid checked for urate crystals. To avoid further attacks, consider changes in living habits.

Among the risk factors are family history suggesting a genetic predisposition and all foods that increase blood urate. Best not to eat liver, kidney, sweetbreads, small fish and the skin of chicken. Eat daily only small amounts, say no more than 150 g, of shellfish, roe, meat, mushrooms, peas or beans. Note that the risk is increased by obesity, high blood pressure, diabetes and heart disease. Avoid beer, it contains purines that increase blood urate. Wine and spirits are less dangerous (Richette and Bardin 2010).

A good idea is to drink liberal amounts of water. This helps the body to remove urate more rapidly. But beware of drinking too much. Part III advises on this. Drink only a little or not at all beverages with high acid content. Acidity opposes the excretion of urate. Many soft drinks are highly acidic (*Table 4*). The lower the pH, the higher the risk.

Table 4. Approximate pH values for some drinks	
Lime juice	2.00 - 2.35
Grapefruit juice	2.90 - 3.25
Apple juice	3.35 - 4.00
Grape juice, canned	3.4
Orange juice	3.00 - 4.00
Cider	3.00 - 4.00
Wine, natural	3.00 - 4.00
Beer	4.50 - 5.50
Coffee	4.50 - 5.50
Tea	5.50 or more
Milk	5.50 or more
Water	5.50 or more

Acidity can be decreased by ingesting alkaline substances. Baking soda, aka bicarbonate, does the job. The usual dose is 2- 6 g (2.5 - 7.5 milliliters) twice a day, fully dissolved in 4 - 8 oz of water. Do not use it for many consecutive days without medical advice. It contains natrium just like salt does and may thus increase blood pressure. Overdose can lead into alkalosis and need for hospital treatment. If self-help is not enough, your doctor can consider the need for long-term drug treatment to decrease the urate level.

18 Aggression and violence-The devil within

Violence is usually brought about by strong aggressive and angry emotions. Most people can control these emotions without resorting to violent acts in normal life. But almost everyone has a boiling point in extreme situations. Causal paths to violence are many and often difficult to identify. Individual risk factors include fairly stable traits of risk-taking and impulsivity as well as paranoid thoughts, need to intimidate or oppress, extreme levels of testosterone, anabolic steroids and some illicit drugs. At the small group level, risk factors may include defamation and the perceived need to behave according to the norms of the peer group. At the societal level, economic distress, cultural conventions and suggestive mass hysteria can play a role.

Hereditary tendency to aggression and maltreatment in childhood may lead into poor executive control of behavior in the mind, followed by impulsive behavior and heavy alcohol intake. The latter may further diminish executive control, by direct effect on the brain or by head trauma. There is an increased risk of becoming violent or becoming a victim of violence. Such persons may behave like small children who have little or no ability to control their aggression. Imagine what it would be like to live with an alcoholic who has toddler's brain, adult size and the strength of a body builder. Frightening, is it not? Maybe the tyrant Pittacus (640 ~ 568

BC) had this in mind when he legislated double punishment for crimes committed while intoxicated. Not without reason was he called one of the seven wise men of ancient Greece.

The role of alcohol in violence varies between individuals. Some people, but not all, loose their self-control easily, especially when intoxicated. An increase in population alcohol consumption does not always lead in a rise in violence. No change or even a decrease has also been observed (Herttua 2011).

Aggressive behavior depends on culture

The relation between aggression and alcohol varies by time and culture. Japanese men drink in groups to decrease tensions due to strict workplace hierarchy. They show practically no aggression (Benedict 1967). Among the Bolivian Camba group drinking also serves to relieve aggression. *"The Camba had weekly benders with laboratory-proof alcohol, and, Dwight Heath said, "There was no social pathology—none. No arguments, no disputes, no sexual aggression, no verbal aggression. There was pleasant conversation or silence." ... "The drinking didn't interfere with work," Heath went on. "It didn't bring in the police. And there was no alcoholism, either."* (Drinking games 2010). Historical documents abound with descriptions of the changing patterns of drinking and aggression, too many to be reviewed here.

Because so many other factors than drinking influence the risk of alcohol-related problems of aggression and violence, it is impossible to estimate any meaningful risk ratios or attributable risks. Instead, the proportion of cases related to alcohol are often cited in the professional journals. This, of course, is not evidence of risk. The proponents do not seem to understand that the logic is false. If you are alarmed to find that 20 % of all road traffic accidents are related to alcohol, you should be more alarmed that 80 % of all road traffic accidents are related to abstinence.

19 Traffic accidents - Drinkers drive better

Waiting for a solution - the self-driving car.

Drinkers are better drivers than abstainers if they do not have alcohol in the body while driving. However, the risk of traffic accident is increased by being enough under the influence of alcohol while driving a car. So what is enough? It is dictated by law.

Tiny amounts of alcohol have no appreciable effect on perception and coordination of movements. In simulator experiments, performance errors arise when blood alcohol level exceeds 0.02 %. Such experiments are more taxing than driving under normal conditions and reveal even minute errors. The risk of road accidents seems to increase when blood alcohol is 0.05 % or more. This increase is directly related to the blood alcohol level. Between the level of 0.05 - 0.1 % the risk of accident is on average 3-fold and at the level of 0.1 % approximately 9-fold. These are crude estimates from case-control and cohort studies. These studies have not been able to control for all other relevant factors that influence the risk. The risk is higher when blood alcohol is rising than when it is falling. Tolerance to alcohol plays a role. The risk is increased by darkness, bad weather, bad road conditions, other traffic, driving speed, fatigue, and by some drugs. Fatigue and alcohol reinforce each other's effect but we do not know how much because there is no reliable method to measure fatigue (Akerstedt et al. 2008). Nor do we have any feasible and accurate method to measure the impairment of driving ability by alcohol. We have to do with a reasonably reliable indicator, blood alcohol, or with a less reliable indicator of the latter, breath alcohol.

The first breath-analyzers were developed in 1927. They were first marketed to housewives so that they could check whether the husband could be allowed to enter home. At present, they are used to screen drivers suspected of being intoxicated since because they are easy to use in the field. But accuracy is less than perfect. Cheap breath-analyzers are unreliable. The police have highly accurate devices (Jones and Andersson 2003). Still, if the device reading disagrees clearly with the driver's memory it is better to conduct also a blood test. The ratio of blood to expiratory air alcohol concentration has been found to have a coefficient of variation between 9 - 19 % (Norberg et al. 2003).

The Grand Rapids Study is the classic, most influential report in this field. A major finding in the original study was the famous dip - drivers with blood alcohol above zero but below 0.05 % had lower accident risk than sober drivers. Otherwise, the higher the blood alcohol, the higher the risk of accident. Later, the picture changed when data were stratified by the usual alcohol intake of the drivers. In every intake group, the accident risk increased in direct proportion to blood alcohol level. No dip was observed. However, among those driving in sober condition, the higher the customary alcohol intake the lower the risk. And the more the customary intake, the less steep was the increase of risk. Among drivers with no alcohol in the blood, with the relative risk for abstainers set at one, the relative risk of daily drinkers was 0.37 (Hurst et al. 1994). This was discovered in 1966 but is not generally known. On the contrary, the findings have been hidden in the literature by graphical manipulation suggesting that the risks at zero level were identical and exaggerating the increase of risk (Edwards et al. 1994 p. 58) as Alfred Uhl has later pointed out (Uhl 2009).

For obvious reasons, randomized trials of legal blood alcohol limit laws are not feasible. We only have before and after studies and cross-regional ones. Some have found significant decreases in traffic accidents (Desapriya and Iwase 1998, Smith 1988, Hingson et al. 2000), others no decrease (Desapriya et al. 2007) or even an increase (Bernhoft and Behrensdorff 2003). Decreasing the legal BAC limit from 0.05 % to 0.03 % did not have any notable association with traffic crashes in Japan (Desapriya et al. 2007).

The above studies are subject to several biases, like changes in criminal activities, drug addictions, drunken comportment, moral attitudes, citizen activism and transportation needs. When several types of actions to decrease drunken driving are introduced during the same period of time, it is impossible to isolate the impact of one of these actions.

131

20 Harms to the unborn - Is there a safe drinking level and what are the causes of fetal alcohol syndrome

Precautionary principle is perhaps good in this case, but moral panic certainly bad.

Alcoholic beverages may harm the unborn child. Suggestive scientific evidence of this was first published in France in the 1960's. It was found that out of the 127 newborn children, 25 had facial or other anomalies. Of the 69 mothers, 54 were alcoholics. The number of alcoholic mothers among the 25 children with anomalies was not reported. Conclusions were based on clinical impression (Lemoine et al. 1968). Similar clinical case reports on the children of alcoholic mothers were published in 1973 and 1974. In 1973, a combination of associated findings was given the name fetal alcohol syndrome, FAS for short. A more appropriate name would have been fetal alcoholism syndrome.

After constructing the diagnosis, the problem gradually became generally known and total abstinence during pregnancy was put forward (The Lancet 1983). As often happens, milder and milder combinations of abnormalities have been given diagnostic labels. These go under the umbrella fetal alcohol spectrum disorder, or FASD. FASD is not meant to be used as a clinical diagnosis. Instead, there are many specific labels in this diagnostic rainbow, such as the acronyms pFAS, FAE, ARND and ARBD, understood only by the select few. There have been and still are many different descriptive rules, known as criteria, to make FAS and FASD diagnoses. Originally, the major criterion for FAS was confirmed heavy alcohol exposure during pregnancy. "Heavy" was never clearly specified. Thus, all pregnant mothers were under suspicion. Even non-drinkers could be suspected of denying their alcohol use. Later, alcohol use during pregnancy was altogether dropped from some diagnostic criteria. There is a lack of studies on the relation between alcohol intake and the risk of FAS. There has been little interest to find out what kind of alcohol intake during pregnancy is harmful although the question is of great practical importance to families where women drink. Fortunately, we can approach the question by deconstructing FAS. We will study the relation between alcohol intake and FAS components separately. The three components are facial and other anomalies, growth deficit and central nervous system abnormalities.

Facial and other anomalies

Congenital anomalies are also called malformations, dysmorphic features or abnormalities. Finding them suggest birth defects or congenital disorders. One meta-analysis focused on facial and brain anomalies thought to be alcohol-related. It combined data on over 130,000 newborn. There was

133

no difference in the incidence of anomalies between abstaining mothers and mothers with an alcohol intake of 24 - 168 g/week (Polygenis et al. 1998).

Growth deficit

Before the FAS risk became generally known, a large cohort of over 9,000 mothers reported on their alcohol intake during the first three months of pregnancy in 1963 - 1969. There were no differences between intake groups below the level of 35 g/day in the birth weight, adjusted for the duration of pregnancy (Kaminski et al. 1978). A later meta-analysis found that 12 g/day or less was not related to the birth weight or to premature birth (Henderson et al. 2007). One study found that premature births were not significantly more common at the intake level of 24 - 168 g/week compared with abstaining (Makarechian et al. 1998). For low birthweight, preterm birth and small for gestational age, a dose-response relation has been found, showing increased risk with heavy use and no risk with light use (Patra et al. 2011).

Central nervous system abnormalities

Although the diagnostic rules talk about central nervous system abnormalities, many studies in fact focus on the statistical distributions of psychological abilities. For example, a meta-analysis of nine studies focused on the total score of the Bailey Scales of Infant Development. This index combines test results on motor, language and cognitive performance. No material differences were found between children born to mothers who abstained or consumed alcohol during pregnancy. In European studies, scores were better among children of drinking mothers than abstaining ones, while in American studies there was no difference (Testa et al. 2003). In Great Britain it was found that, compared with never-drinkers, intake of 8 - 16 g/week during pregnancy was followed by better cognitive ability among boys at the age of three years. The boys were more mature and showed less hyperactivity or conduct problems. The boys to mothers with an intake of 48 g or more per occasion had more emotional problems. There were no differences at all among girls. Findings were similar at the age of five and seven years (Kelly et al. 2013; Kelly et al. 2012; Kelly et al. 2009). This agrees with findings from other studies (Testa et al. 2003; Falgreen et al. 2012; Larroque et al. 1995; Larroque and Kaminski 1998).

Risk level

Based on the available studies it seems that 20 - 30 g/day during pregnancy does not harm the fetus. The risk will be lower if consumption pace is slow and the pregnant mother does not have risk factors that strengthen the effect of alcohol. However, rapid gulping may be dangerous and higher intake seems certainly risky. The risk level is a population average, good advice for most mothers but not for those who differ much from the average. It is not an absolutely safe level. It is

135

better to abstain completely if the pregnant woman worries or easily suffers from feelings of guilt or anxiety because of drinking. Social pressure may influence your decision.

Some researchers argue that no risk level can be detected (Streissguth et al. 2004). Well, if you fit to your data a statistical model that presumes a continuous relation with no threshold then you cannot see any threshold. Other researchers argue that if any guidelines advise on a risk limit this would make some pregnant women drink more than the limit. They require strict abstinence although their own studies have not found any problems at the intake level of 70 g/week or 1- 2 drinks occasionally (O'Leary and Bower 2012; O'Leary et al. 2010; May et al. 2008). Guidelines should be based on scientific findings, not on moralistic views.

Causes of fetal alcohol syndrome and related diagnoses

The early FAS studies focused on mothers with severe alcoholism. Alcoholics' risk factor profile differs from the average in many ways. Some more recent studies have tried to ascertain other risk factors. Among the poor in South Africa, heavy drinking and poor nutrition is common. One study found that FAS and partial FAS were associated with small body size (probably due to nutritional deficiencies), low income, education and social group as well as smoking. Moreover, intoxication during pregnancy (estimated blood alcohol 0.1 - 0.2 %) was a risk factor (May et al. 2008). Other risk factors, found in other studies, include stress, high lead levels, high maternal age, prenatal exposure to cocaine or cannabis, paternal drinking and drug use at the time of pregnancy (Sood et al. 2001; Archer 2011). Having one FAS child increases the FAS risk for later offspring. This and the finding that one of twins can have FAS but the other not suggest that genes play a role (Golden 2005). Alcoholic mothers with several risk factors and social problems are the risk group in desperate need of help. Putting the blame on moderate users brings no gain. Nevertheless, blaming the innocent has become popular.

Panic, politics and warning labels

After inventing the diagnosis, fetal alcohol exposure was turned into a major public health problem in the USA. The focus changed from the hardships of alcoholic mothers to light drinkers among women of fertile age. Moral panic brought about political action. In 1981, the Surgeon General warned that pregnant women and those considering pregnancy (!) should not drink alcoholic beverages. In 1989 it was legislated that every bottle should carry a label stating that "According to the Surgeon General, women should not drink alcoholic beverages during pregnancy because of the risk of birth defects". This brought about anxiety in some women prone to worry who made the mistake of having an occasional drink. In contrast, the intended effects of warning labels on the bottles were found to be materially nonexistent (Stockwell 2006). The

137

number of newborn FAS children continued to increase (Golden 2005)). Judicial abuse of the diagnostic labels was discovered. Arguing that a crime or misdemeanor was due to prenatal alcohol exposure sometimes brought about more lenient sentences. Messages were contradictory. On one hand, avoid alcohol consumption during pregnancy; on the other hand, do not become unnecessarily alarmed about an occasional drink. The panic has spread worldwide.

138

VI

ALCOHOLISM - THE RAGE TO ENJOY

Only good things can be abused.

A homeless Indian sees his grandmother's regalia in the window of a pawnshop and wants to buy it. He does not have the money. The kind-hearted pawnbroker promises to sell the regalia with no profit if the Indian comes back within 24 hours. He even gives the man 20 dollars start-up money. Now the task is to find the rest of the 1000 dollars. A difficult task, but Jackson Jackson (known also as Jackson squared) tries hard. With some luck he earns some money, but always spends it on food and drinks, mostly on huge amounts of booze, for his friends and for himself. Late in the night he is buying shots of bad whisky, when at 2 a.m. the barman shouts: "Closing time!" At that hour a few Indians are "still drinking hard after a long, hard day of drinking ". So wrote Sherman Alexie in *What you pawn I will redeem* (Alexie 2005). It is a compassionate and magical short story.

A brilliant surgeon, admired by his colleagues, staff and patients, famous for his operating skills, international clientele and effective fund raising for a charitable cancer fund has a secret. He drinks, beats his wife, daughter and dog. He likes his breakfast orange juice laced with vodka. So wrote his daughter in her autobiography (Dickson Wright 2007).

The bootlegger George Cassiday confessed in a newspaper that he had sold liquor during Prohibition to a

141

majority of both Houses of Congress and the typical customer had a capacity of two or three quarts a week, tells a history of the Prohibition in the USA (Okrent 2010).

What do these storied men share? They come from the opposite ends of social strata, but all had very heavy alcohol intake. The first one does not seem to control his craving, the second his aggression, of the rest we have no additional information. Were these men alcoholics? What is alcoholism and what are its causes?

Alcoholism, aka alcohol dependence, aka alcohol addiction, is another fuzzy concept. It escapes rigorous definition. Fuzzy concepts can be useful in everyday communication as approximate signs of direction but do not take us far.

Alcoholism belongs to the class of addictions. The alcoholic is too much attached to drinking. Just like some other people are strongly attached to eating, smoking, coffee, drugs, sex, gambling, shopping, exercise, sunbathing, work, power, some significant other person or something else. One carrot addict is known according to a case report in the journal *Addiction*.

In addictions, there is excess in the search for enjoyment, a desire that is difficult to quench and dejection afterwards. A few addictions are not harmful, many are. The more harms the addiction brings about, the more likely it is considered to be a bad habit or a disease. A person susceptible to one addiction is likely to be susceptible to others, too. Alcoholism can be substituted by gambling, gambling by sex and so on. Self-help and professional treatment are mostly based on similar principles whatever the type of addiction. If the attachment is strong but harmless we do not call it a disease. The rich who have an art collection addiction are not coerced into treatment. However, they may go to jail if the are caught contracting thieves to supply them with the items desired. I will argue that the biomedical definitions of alcoholism are just old ideas disguised in new jargon. They maintain untenable assumptions on the cause of alcoholism. To find out the causal paths we need to look elsewhere. However, the old ideas stay alive since they serve various vested interests. One of the latter is the powerful alcoholism treatment industry. It promises cure, but there is no clear evidence.

21 The disease concept

Is pleasure a disease? No, but it can bring about addictions.

It seems that it was English priests who launched the idea of alcoholism as a disease in the 17th century (Heyman 2009). Medical men of the Enlightenment, Thomas Trotter (1760 ~ 1832) in Scotland and Benjamin Rush (1745 ~ 1813) in North America supported this view. It was spread further by the Alcoholics Anonymous (AA), born in 1934 in the USA. Academic alcohol research was based on early AA ideas, starting from the 1940's. Elvin Morton Jellinek (1890 ~ 1963) described the characteristics and the "typical" course of alcoholism. Alcoholism was seen as a compulsive disease. There was craving that leads to the inability to abstain and loss of control that leads to the inability to stop drinking. The only cure to this condition was complete abstinence. This removed the harms by not the desire. Once an alcoholic, always an alcoholic. These ideas have continued to shape our present diagnostic descriptions of all addictions, now called dependence or dependency. Diagnostic criteria for alcohol dependence rely mainly on descriptions of behavior. In the DSM-IV by the American Psychiatric Association, there are seven items. Two of these, tolerance and withdrawal, can also be sometimes measured objectively, although this is seldom feasible and never necessary. The presence of three out of the seven items suffice for diagnosis. Five of the criteria depend on the assessment and interpretation of behavior, being

1. a great deal of time is spent in activities necessary to obtain alcohol, use alcohol or recover from its effects
2. important social, occupational, or recreational activities are given up or reduced because of alcohol use
3. alcohol use is continued despite knowledge of having a physical or psychological problem that is likely to have been exacerbated by alcohol
4. alcohol is often taken in larger amounts or over a longer period than was intended
5. persistent desire or unsuccessful efforts to cut down or control alcohol abuse

The order of criteria in the above list differs from the original in order to better see the similarity between the past and the current formulations. Criteria 1- 3 can be interpreted as attempts to map out craving and criteria 4 and 5 to enfold loss of control to stop drinking. The underlying interpretation seems to be that if drinking is routinely repeated, this implies strong desire, in other words craving, and if drinking goes on longer than originally planned, this is evidence of loss of control.

Criterion 3 hints that alcoholism can bring about health and social problems. In practice, it might be an important feature. Alcoholism (and other substance addictions) often undermine work ability, social competence and healthy leisure activities. This an essential feature of addictions, as Gene M. Heyman has pointed out (Heyman 2009). They are antisocial behaviors. Other passions work contrariwise or are harmless.

The criteria in DSM-IV are practically identical to the international ICD-10. The item content in the latter is similar except that there is one item less because criteria 1 and 2 in the above list have been joined into one criterion. The new DSM-5 has similar criteria, only the number of items has been expanded to 11. Diagnostic criteria need to be repeatedly changed, so that they may remain the same. One of the effects of changing criteria is that the diagnostic entity is becoming more and more heterogeneous. The DSM-IV criteria allowed for 99 different combinations. The new DSM-V allows for 2036 combinations to alcohol use disorder, the current entity (Edenberg and McClintick 2018).

The diagnostic systems are vague on cutoff of the criteria. It is not possible to make a clear distinction between who meets the criteria and who does not. Thus, the diagnosis depends on the skill, consistency and subjective preferences of the professional. Wide leeway is possible. Think about the fictional character Jackson Jackson, the homeless Indian we met in the beginning of this chapter. He seems to fulfill easily the behavioral criteria of alcoholism. The surgeon would most likely have been protected from the alcoholism label because of his profession, fame and success in his medical career, even if the battered family members had thought otherwise. The congressmen drinking three quarts a week during Prohibition were probably alcoholics or at least heavy drinkers in the evenings and temperance zealots in the daytime. The fuzziness of the diagnosis is not merely due to lack of rules for cutoffs. It may be that there are no natural cutoffs. Early pondering saw the dependence syndrome to exist in degrees (Edwards et al. 1977). Now the brand new DSM-5 has reinvented this idea and sees the possibility that there are several degrees of alcoholism.

Disease as a social construction

Alcoholism is a real problem but the disease concept may be seen as a social construction. In that, it is similar to several other disease constructions. Drapetomania, the compulsive desire of slaves to run away, used to be prevalent in the USA before the Civil War. Europe experienced a long epidemic of witchcraft between 1500 - 1750. Homosexuality was highly esteemed in ancient Greece, later considered a crime, then a disease and now it is in many countries normal, if not fashionable. Some detriments have a weak status as diseases. They have little in common with those entities that are seen to be proper diseases by most experts and other members of society. There is no consensus whether these problems are diseases or not. Only a difference of opinions. For example, from the psychological viewpoint one could legitimately claim that alcoholism is a bad habit because one way to understand it is a routine in the habit loop (Duhigg 2012). There is no way to award the disease status logically because there is no clear general definition of disease against which alcoholism can be

147

compared.

Once widely accepted, social constructions continue to persist until they are dropped. What is usually called for is that science finds evidence that proves the construction false or true. It would be easier to accept the disease concept of alcoholism if there were some specific brain defect or dysfunction, or at least some risk factor that would predict with good precision who will become an alcoholic and who will not. There is no such evidence. Yet, the disease concept remains popular. In USA, for example, alcoholism was considered a disease by 20 % of the population in 1946, but by 90 % in the 1990's (Golden 2005). Why the popularity? One partial explanation has been presented.

Addicts bring out fear and rejection in other people, just like evil spirits and witches earlier. This may be due to the fact that the addict has consciously rejected the norms and rules of society. Instead, the addict has chosen pleasure, leisure, laziness and freedom. There is one type of alcoholic that fits this description. In this case, the overwhelming aim is drinking. Everything else serves this target. Time is spent in getting booze, finding drinking companions, and improving the economic and health preconditions for drinking, for example in treatment. However, there are also other types of alcoholics.

The existence of the lazy alcoholic cannot be accepted. The addict is viewed as a traitor (Blum 1969). Since we do no longer believe in the existence of witches, some other more plausible explanation must be found. It must convince us that the addict has no free will. Rather, he or she is under the spell of a disease due to an evil substance. Enter brain research. Only the expert can understand and interpret the results of hi-tech brain research. Only an expert could criticize this research (but why would he or she rock the boat?). The public is dependent on the expert opinion. Slogans such as "dependence is a chronic brain disease" and "drugs hijack the pleasure pathway" sell well. Money for brain research, fake justification for the treatment industry and liberation from responsibility for the addict are delivered. The dark side of the disease concept is that it increases stigma and discrimination (Schomerus et al. 2011). Fuzzy diagnosis bears hard consequences.

22 Biomedical views on the cause of addiction

Much ado about weak effects in practice.

There is little new in the current biomedical models of alcoholism. The central concepts remain the same. The current diagnostic descriptions reflect the concepts of craving, compulsion, inability to abstain and the loss of control of drinking. The same lack of progress shows for causal assumptions. The ideas on the causes of addictions have, however, been modified to fit into the dominant scientific ideas of the day. No longer is the cause thought to be an allergy as AA used to believe. Now the key is the brain, but this is no news. Already in the 19th century, the then fashionable Keeley's cure claimed that the treatment provided recovery from the irresistible craving of nerve cells for alcohol (Okrent 2010). Currently, there are two main beliefs on the causes. The first assumes that the cause precedes alcoholism and is found in the genes. The second believes that long-term use of alcohol changes the way the brain works. Alcohol hijacks the brain, goes the sales punch line.

The role of genes is exaggerated

The media and the scientific community like to overstate the role of genes. Genes do play a role but a small one. At present about 1500 genes associated with addictions are known but these genes take part also in a multitude of life-sustaining processes in the body. What often happens is that a group of scientists collects a small sample and finds an association between alcoholism and one gene or other. The media report that the gene for addiction has been finally found. Later, much larger samples or meta-analyses of several smaller ones are unable to confirm the finding. This removes the topic's news value.

The exaggerated belief seems to be supported by two things. First, a considerable minority of Oriental people (20 – 40 %) have a deficiently functioning enzyme system due to genetic makeup. It slows the breakdown of alcohol in the body and causes unpleasant symptoms while drinking (Kalant 2010). However, this pertains to a minority of the world's population, and it does not predispose to alcoholism. On the contrary, it protects from heavy drinking.

Secondly, the meaning of the heritability coefficient is commonly misunderstood. It is true that these coefficients are fairly large for alcoholism. It is often said that the coefficients show that genes explain about 50 % of alcoholism. However, the heritability coefficient does not take into account the interaction between genes and environment (Rose 2005). If the population attributable fraction is calculated by state-of-the-art epidemiologic methods, as is commonly done for diseases, the share of genes in explaining alcoholism is approximately 8 %.

151

The above calculation is based on the following premises: Parental history is an indicator of the effect of genes. Among the children of alcoholics the risk of becoming an alcoholic is twofold compared with other children (Poikolainen 2005). The birth rate among alcoholics is equal to that among other parents. The 12-month prevalence of alcoholism is 3.8 % (Hasin et al. 2007). The result overstates the role of genes because some part of the parental risk is likely to be due to drinking while pregnant and some other part to early child-rearing practices.

The false step of the animal experiment

Animal experiments to find the biological basis of addiction have been going on for more than 60 years. No breakthrough has yet been made. Normally, animals do not drink alcoholic beverages voluntarily. To overcome this, two rat models were bred, one strain preferring alcohol and another shunning alcohol (Sarviharju et al. 2004). Much high-level research has been done although the model is not good for alcoholism. The consumption level was similar between the strains among the male rats. Among female rats there was but a small difference. The rats preferring alcohol were actually moderate drinkers - average blood alcohol was 0.036 % and maximal level 0.115 % (Rintala et al. 1997). No withdrawal symptoms were observed after 18 months of continuous alcohol exposure (Rintala et al. 1998). The strain preferring alcohol had longer life-span than the rats shunning alcohol (Sarviharju et al. 2004).

Laboratory animals live caged in confined environment, far from their natural habitat. This is likely to produce stress and abnormal behavior. In contrast, rats raised in social colonies and enriched environment behave more normally and only a few become extreme over-consumers of alcohol. The latter few show a variety of alterations in behavior, including chronic inactivity and low dominance standing (Ellison & Potthoff 1984). Isolated mice have the highest ethanol preference (Holgate et al. 2017).

Animal experiments hold out little promise. The neurobiological studies on the rat and other animals can shed light on the general workings of neural cells in the rat brain but not on addictions, since the neural processes are similar for both addictions and other behaviors (Kalant 2010).

The tenets of the present biomedical models have been proven wrong

In alcoholism, there is no obvious inability to abstain or loss of control of drinking. Studies on several thousands of people found that most cases with a diagnosis of alcohol dependence were mild and recovered without any treatment, and a good deal of these were able to drink moderately later (Dawson et al. 2005; Heyman 2009 p. 69-79). Experiments have shown that the alcoholic can take drinks containing alcohol without losing the control of drinking (Fingarette 1988 p. 35-41). Thus, there is no innate inability to abstain and no absolute loss of control. The tenets of the disease concept do not hold. However, there

153

seems to be a dislike to abstain and not much interest in controlling drinking. The strong claim has been refuted but a weak characterization of the problem makes more sense. Except the word "disease". Diseases do not reward, alcoholism does.

If the tenets work in recovery, the effect is psychological. Beliefs can guide behavior. Strong beliefs may strengthen the will to put into practice a major decision. Such great decisions are called conversion (Ullman-Margalit 2006). A vivid example of the conversion from wordly pleasures to the spiritual realm is the life of Saint Francis of Assisi (de la Bedoyere 1962). In such a situation, a person sees that a major change is necessary and there is no other way. A conversion is a way to redeem the sins and do away with the shame. Adopting totally new values is a spiritual rebirth. This one of the central tenets in the AA ideology. There is much practical wisdom in AA which plays a crucial role in the lives of those people benefiting from it. Some of it is ancient, already evident in the teachings of the ancient Greek and Roman philosophers, Democritus, Epicurus, Seneca and Marcus Aurelius among others. The Serenity Prayer,

God, grant me the serenity
to accept the things I cannot change,
Courage to change the things I can,
And wisdom to know the difference.

coined by the theologian Reinhold Niebuhr, has the same idea as what the Stoic Epictetus (50 ~ 135 AD) some 2,000 years

154

ago taught. We can change our mental faculties: beliefs, impulses, desires, and aversions, while our position in the world is largely beyond our powers of influence, such as the behavior of our fellow people, our financial possessions, glory and social status. Peace of mind can be achieved with self-control, decency, modesty, dignity and moderation. He even advised that "When you have learned to nourish your body frugally, do not pique yourself upon it; nor, if you drink water, be saying upon every occasion, "I drink water." (Epictetus 1948). Meaning, do not boast that you are an abstainer (or a drinker for that matter, I'd like to add).

23 From general principles to risk factors

Almost everything is risky, but predictive power is impractically small.

There are many attempts to explain alcoholism, but no coherent theory has emerged that could be either confirmed or falsified (West 2006). Alcoholism is a slippery concept. What do we really know about alcoholism? Very little. On average, alcoholics are as intelligent as other people. Cognitive and executive functions have been similar among addicts compared with their non-addict twins (Heyman 2009 p. 151). There seem to be as many kinds of alcoholics as other people. Mark Keller (1907 ~ 1995) was deeply versed in the subject. He quipped "in alcoholism everything that one measures is either increased or decreased" and "alcoholics differ from each other as much as non-alcoholics. They all show, however, one common factor: they all take alcoholic drink." But the question is how they drink.

Participant observations, as noted earlier in chapter 3, have shown that alcoholics may typically consume between 350 to 470 g/day if there are no serious restrictions to the availability of the drink. Assuming that they underestimate their intake as much as all others, their reported intake might be roughly between 100 and 200 g/day. Such figures are actually often reported in research articles.

There seems to be something extraordinary in the way how alcoholics take their drinks. They differ from other heavy drinkers by having fewer days of abstinence, more days of heavy drinking, higher frequency of intoxicating drinking and atypical temporal drinking patterns (Dawson 2000a; Dawson 2000b). Alcoholics have been found to have more occasions of intoxication and eye-opener drinks in hangover than marital status- and age-adjusted controls (Bruun and Markkanen 1961).

Some argue that any alcohol use starts the primrose path to alcoholism. In contrast to this, there seems to be a threshold. In Denmark, it was found that the occurrence of alcoholism over a 25-year follow-up time increased significantly only among men having more than 22-41 drinks weekly (Flensborg-Madsen et al. 2007). The comparison group was those drinking less than one drink weekly. Smoking was independently associated with the risk of alcoholism.

Let us see if we can explain at least a small part of the occurrence of alcoholism with the general principles of human behavior and from the various particular conditions that we will call risk factors. There are two kinds of the latter, external strong temptations and internal weaknesses that undermine resistance to the former. Think of Odysseus passing the island of Sirens. The Siren song was an irresistible invitation but prevented by bee-wax in the ears and bindings to the mast.

157

Voluntary choices

We humans have in our conscious brain a slow but rational and logical decision-making system. This is the basis of free will (Rolls 2012). Economic theory assumes that we use it when making decisions and carrying them out. A decision is always reached by calculating the utilities and choosing the action with the highest utility. The principle of utility calculation was explained at the beginning of Part IV.

In the simplest case, you compare one reward and one punishment here and now. The reward wins. Almost as simple as that is a comparison of two rewards, the highest utility wins. If drinking consistently gets the highest utility value, then you will drink. The highest score may be due to the reward given by, say, good taste, euphoric feeling or drinking companions. It may be due to the promise of these things. Some people find kinky things rewarding (Kalant 2010; Ainslie 2001 p. 59). This is difficult to understand for the majority of people who would find the same rewards averse.

Things get slightly more complicated if you compare the expected values of future rewards, and the smaller reward is available sooner than the bigger reward. The rational mind says that you should always prefer the greater reward even if it takes longer to attain. In this case, you are consistent in your preferences. Mathematically, you are discounting exponentially future utility. However, we humans and other mammals are not always consistent decision-makers. Our preferences can change. This is perhaps due to the unconscious, more primitive, genetically determined and emotionally guided decision-making system that relies on stimuli and reinforcement. Or it can be due to the crude rules of thumb (heuristics in the trade jargon) that we often rely on in rapid decision-making (Slovic et al. 1981; Slovic 1987; Casey et al. 2011). Even if we have decided always to prefer the option with the highest future utility, our preferences can be reversed. If the goal with the highest utility is to be achieved later in future than the alternative lower utility, this reversal can take place when the Siren song of the alternative smaller utility comes close enough to be heard. Mathematically, you are discounting hyperbolically the future utility. A good deal of experimental evidence supports this view (Ainslie 2001).

Take two tennis players, Bob and Tom. On Monday, Bob decides that because he wants to beat Tom in their Sunday match he needs to be in pristine condition and must avoid Saturday reveling. However, on Saturday afternoon the utility of the evening drinking party exceeds the utility of victory over Tom. The primitive mind whispers to Bob: go and party, there is enough man in you to beat Tom anyway. But after the Sunday match has been lost Bob is recanting. His rational mind might try to rescue the damage done by the false decision by inventing some pretext that will soothe ego's regret. Humans are good at inventing excuses.

Consider another case of changing preferences. Let us say that you can repeatedly choose either A or B. Initially you like A more than B, but having it a few times it loses so much of its appeal that now B is preferred. After having B a few times the preferences again switch. Experimental evidence and decision-making tests show that this is common. Some important conclusions follow. First, the option that has more appeal at present will usually be chosen. Secondly, this leads to over-consumption. Thirdly, this brings about fewer benefits than a strategy considering choices as a set of many instead only one at present (Heyman 2009).

Addictions do not only reward but also punish. If harms arise or are expected, it is time to weigh the reward against the punishment. Again, a rational decision-maker will choose the option with the highest utility. Rational choice is most difficult when the rewards are close to you in future but the punishments far away. It is difficult to estimate the probabilities of far-way states and easy to overestimate what you can get here and now. Alcoholics facing harm are often in this situation. It is called ambivalence. At the same time, the alcoholic wants to drink and be saved from the harms of the drink. When asked what is their concept of moderate drinking, some alcoholics said after considerable mental effort: It would be drinking two bottles of vodka every day without any detriments at all.

The choice switches easily from the goal that would have been the best in the long term to the choice that produces immediate reward when the temptation is at hand. Ambivalence explains why the alcoholic clearly understands and accepts the need to stop drinking when in treatment but easily relapses when in a wet environment. The enjoyment is followed by bittersweet recanting. Being an alcoholic is like being lovesick. William Shakespeare (1564? ~ 1616) knew this well when he wrote

> *Enjoyed no sooner but despised straight;*
> *Past reason hunted; and no sooner had,*
> *Past reason hated, as a swallowed bait,* [11]

Perhaps he had read Epictetus. This philosopher advised the ancient Greeks and Romans to take care to not being carried away when thinking about some pleasure, First wait, then think about two things: the moment of experiencing this pleasure and at moment when the enjoyment ends and you recant and blame yourself. Then think how pleased you could be if you had quelled the desire.

Willpower

In general, several practices may strengthen the will to stick to the greater long-term utility and shun the temptation of the smaller but sooner available one. It may help to make rules, allow no exceptions to the rules and think that all your choices are a part of a larger program. The latter underlines the idea that one slip once may endanger the whole plan. It is dangerous to think that an exception can be made today if only the rule is

---

[11]   part of Sonnet CXXIX, www.shakespeares-sonnets.com

observed in future (Ainslie 2001). Think that the future is being decided now. Social support, rituals and pledges may help. All organizations that aim at social cohesion use these means. Consider armies, political parties, religions, AA or the mafia. Even families partly resort to these means. One part of willpower may be innate, perhaps genetic. This is suggested by the marshmallow experiment by Walter Mischel where differences were observed in willpower between children aged four years. When the temptation presents itself, try either to involve your mind with something else, whatever might interest you, or give the temptation a less seductive mental image. Some experimental and follow-up studies suggest that this might work (Casey et al. 2011).

Willpower is in some ways like a muscle. It becomes stronger when you train it. Successful resisting of temptations strengthens the willpower. Following rules for a longer time can replace difficult pondering about what to do through easy routines. If training is too hard and tasks too heavy, willpower will weaken. Mental stress and problems tend to decrease willpower (Holton 2007). If the routine serves your immediate rewards well but is bad for your best long-term interests, then much willpower is needed to break the routine (Fingarette 1988 p. 105). Alcoholism is a state where the willpower is undermined by the rage to enjoy.

Risk factors

A life is like a journey in a jungle with many diverging paths.

162

Moving through this jungle involves both risks and opportunities. It is an advantage to learn from good guides, analyze and consider options, plan ahead, set goals, find means to reach them and learn from mistakes. A brief and simplified sketch of this process relating to intoxicating drinking follows.

Genes and maternal exposures during pregnancy produce newborns with relatively stable temperament patterns. No one knows how many temperament types there are. Different theories suggest from three to nine. Patterns match or mismatch with the temperament of the parents. If these types for the children and parents match well, upbringing is likely to be easy. If not, conflicts and difficulties arise and special education skills for the parents are needed, but there is no clear evidence of effectiveness (Barlow et al. 2006; Barlow et al. 2015; Miller et al. 2011). Temperament types further clash or harmonize at pre-school and school when the child meets other children and teachers. The parents, and increasingly over time, the subject itself can decide which paths to take, avoid or retreat from. In the teen years the peers play an important role. Impulsive and extrovert teens are at higher risk to all kinds of addictions than others in adolescence. Using alcohol and mind-changing drugs is psychologically motivated mainly by sensation-seeking and feeling 'high'. The social and cultural set the background environment that favors or inhibits risk-taking.

First encounters with intoxication are often less than pleasant. This makes some lifelong abstainers. Others continue on, often tempted by older and more experienced buddies. The brain then adapts and the experience becomes desirable. Hangovers can be cured by further use. School performance and relations with elders suffer. Stepping back is possible at all times, easier or more difficult, depending on a multitude of factors.

Adolescents prone to worry, neuroticism, anxiety and depression are more risk-averse than the novelty-seeking ones. Addiction may begin later when motivated by self-medicating bad feelings. Several forms of hardships later in life, like loneliness, divorce, unemployment, or loosing a close friend, may lead into addictions. Indeed, any traumatic event may dispose on to addiction.

Among the best known risk factors for alcoholism are parental history, smoking, impulsivity and other externalizing behavior patterns as well as anxiety and other internalizing behavior patterns (Poikolainen 2005). Many other factors may be involved as well.

Parental history points to genetic, intrauterine and early child-rearing influences. Smoking weakens the effects of alcohol and may thus increase amounts consumed. Impulsive people tend to change their priorities easily (Heyman 2009 p. 158) and are prone to addictions (Bretteville-Jensen 1999; Kalis et al. 2008). Excess impulsivity can be a personality trait. It is also common in many mental disorders, such as conduct disorder, attention-deficit disorder and antisocial personality disorder. People who easily become anxious may start to relieve the tension by alcohol with undue thoroughness.

Anxiety may be a personality trait or a symptom of several mental disorders. Falls and other accidents may damage the executive functions in the brain. This can worsen decision-making ability and willpower.

The risk factors of alcoholism may emerge as early as in childhood or adolescence before any alcohol has been ingested. Both externalizing and internalizing problems degrade school performance and career possibilities. If the future does not promise fulfillment of long-term positive goals, only immediate gratification remains and will push towards crime and addictions. Social contacts and communication as well as cultural attitudes and norms also play a role. Risk factors for heavy alcohol intake episodes in adolescence are similar to the risk factors for alcoholism (Poikolainen 2010). However, there is also much resilience and many options for good development in adolescence.

All of the many risk factors are weak. Somebody may have one risk factor, another several, and still another person a completely different set of risk factors. There are many various pathways to alcoholism. Predicting who will become an alcoholic is difficult. Forecasts fail in most cases.

The bad habit loop

Risk factors are usually something that exert their influence for a long time, both before the onset of alcoholism and during its course. Just like smoking is a risk factor for coronary heart disease and continuing to smoke worsens the course of heart

165

disease. Risk factors seem to indicate heightened susceptibility to drinking cues. Cues are a kind of temptation. In other words, cues are short-acting stimuli that elicit the expectation of reward in the mind. There are myriads of cues in our environment. The stimuli can be either conscious or unconscious.

The expectations initiate behavior aiming to get a reward. Strong expectations (cravings) can sustain this behavior repeatedly even in cases in which many attempts are required to attain the reward. Repetition may turn the behavior into a routine. A habit is then born. If the target of the craving is something that drinking has given, may give again in the future, and the attempt to acquire it requires drinking in alcoholic proportions, then we might say that alcoholism is not a disease but a bad habit.

The control of behavior is an ancient idea. For example, the Greek Stoic philosopher Epictetus taught some 2000 years ago that if you alter your habits and adopt a new practice it will become a habit easy to maintain, the very advice Hamlet told his mother. Nowadays we seem to understand why this may work. One psychological theory says that addiction as well as any other reward-seeking behavior can be understood as a sort of habit loop. In general, a cycle of the loop looks like this: cue → routine → reward.

The routine is repeated as long as the reward is delivered. You can account for almost any behavior with this model. It has been used to explain successes of a brand of toothpaste, winning sports games and recovery from all kinds of addictions. The main tenet is that you cannot alter the cues or the reward. What you can do, however, is to identify the cue → routine → reward pathway and then change the routine (Duhigg 2012). In alcoholism, this presupposes that alcoholic drinking is a routine and thus something else should be found to reward in place of drinking.

To find a routine to replace alcoholism might first require a search for meaningful cues and the reward brought about by alcoholism. Is the reward friendship, company of your fellow man or woman, alleviation of anxiety, altruism or something else? And is the cue anxiety, loneliness, promise of getting high or something else?

If there is only one reward and a few cues, the idea above perhaps works. For example, if the reward is alleviation of anxiety or stress, you might be able to replace drinking by meditation, walking, music or some other activity that relaxes. If cues triggering anxiety are identified, cues might be avoided or relaxation started as a preventive. Any group activity, such as team games, social hobbies or self-help groups may assist if the reward is companionship. If the reward is feeling high, help can be found in exercise, entertainment or daydreaming. Unfortunately, the new reward for ex-alcoholics has often been gambling, drugs or other addictive activities. Another common problem is that heavy drinking is a relatively easy way to attain many different kinds of rewards. In cases where cues and rewards abound, clarification of the loop components seems a

Herculean task. And what if the reward becomes the cue and a vicious circle develops? Then there is big trouble. The finding that alcoholics aim at intoxication and at all hours of the day and night suggests that drinking is the dominant reward in some cases.

"Natural" and self-help recovery

Good friends can be the best medicine.

Many alcoholics recover without any professional treatment. A retrospective survey of a nationally representative sample of US adults aged 18 and over revealed that 75% of subjects with a DSM-IV alcohol dependence diagnosis had recovered, and of these 74.5% had never had any treatment for their dependence (Dawson et al. 2005). What are the causes of such recovery? Faith and fear, to put it bluntly.

Faith in a higher power in heaven, love of a dear one or friends, or your own willpower may help in some cases. Some psychologists call this latter kind of faith self-efficacy. Fear of losing something important, say, a beloved one, friends, job, professional status, money, driver's license or something else might be a decisive factor. The significant reward varies between persons and may be difficult to determine. Let me offer an example.

In a motivational interview, an effort is made clarify the

benefits and harms in the hope that the alcoholic will see the importance of abstaining. One alcoholic had lost his job and his wife had left him. He was told that his liver had lost most of its function. He could care less. He didn't want to see the his wife again, work had been dead boring and he didn't appreciate the value of liver function. He had decided to stop drinking, however, because intoxication hindered him in taking good care of his beloved dog (Leigh 1999). The causes of sobering up can be extraordinary. I know one guy who hopped on the water wagon because he completed his academic PhD thesis. Another sobered up when he saw ants dancing, and he was not a myrmecologist.

Things become difficult if you have nothing to lose. In the end, the alcoholic could be similar to the Drunk alone on a tiny star in the book *The Little Prince* (1943) by Antoine de Saint-Exupéry (1900 ~ 1944). The Prince landed on the star and asked why the Drunk was drinking. "To forget," said he. "To forget what?" "To forget that I am ashamed." "What are you ashamed of?" "I am ashamed that I drink."

169

24 The unknown value of professional treatment

> *If the patient is cured it is because the skill of the therapist, if not, because of the in-curability of the patient's alcoholism.*

There are a great number of studies on the effectiveness of alcoholism treatment. Practically all compare the effects of two or more treatments. If the studies are well-made, small differences, or none at all, are usually found between the treatments compared. These differences are of little practical importance. If the differences are large, an expert is usually able to find biases, such as errors in randomization, patient selection, manipulation of measurements, or inadequate statistical analysis. In the substandard studies, the result usually favors the treatment method of the sponsor. Such studies are shamelessly used in the marketing of professional treatment services. This reminds me of what George Bernard Shaw (1856 ~ 1950) once said, something like: every profession is a conspiracy against the common man.

My main point here is that the effectiveness of alcoholism treatment is and will remain unknown. To learn about its effectiveness we should compare treatment with no treatment. There are no adequate studies on this question.

170

Three were found in a large meta-analysis but none were really about alcoholism (SBU 2001). There is no way to study this question anymore because the common overriding misconception is that any treatment does good. The alcoholism treatment industry would oppose any comparisons with a no-treatment control group by claiming that it would be unethical. If by some blessing such a study were to be carried out, the comparison might be biased. The no-treatment control group would probably suffer from mental distress leading to an inferior outcome since they received no treatment. This is the psychological do-bad effect (nocebo), the opposite of do-good (placebo). Earlier, no such problems were apparent. One early study compared intensive treatment with no treatment at all among 100 alcoholics. No differences in the outcome were found (Orford and Edwards 1977). Randomized placebo-controlled trials on the effect of drugs (acamprosate, baclofen, naltrexone) on the various self-reported drinking outcomes have found none or only minimal positive effect according to the Cochrane reviews and meta-analyses (Rösner et al. 2010a; Rösner et al. 2010b; Minozzi et al. 2018). This is not convincing evidence because self-reports are inaccurate also in this kind of trials (Hämäläinen et al. 2020).

Studies on the mortality of alcoholics after treatment may shed some light on the question of treatment effectiveness. The advantage is that all deaths among all alcoholics can be ascertained. In contrast, when the outcome is sobriety or controlled drinking a large number of alcoholics will be lost to

171

follow-up and their fate remains unknown. When only those whose fate is known are being compared are results usually seriously biased. The worst cases are excluded. Moreover, those who agree to take part in randomized trials are usually milder cases than those who refuse. Commonly, mortality studies compare the number deaths among alcoholics to the number expected on the basis of the entire population mortality rates. Indirectly age- and sex-standardized mortality ratios show the relative risk. Typically, alcoholics have 2-fold to 4-fold higher mortality in large studies (Bruun et al. 1975; Schmidt and de Lint 1970; Edwards et al. 1978; Combs-Orme et al. 1983; Liskow et al. 2000; Laramée et al. 2015). Treatment does not seem to have any large effect on the mortality of alcoholics.

I am not saying that treatment could not help in some cases, at some times, in some situations. All I am saying is that on average treatment does not seem to have any notable effect. Because of this, we might be satisfied with only two kinds of treatment. Treatments should be either be free-of-charge services by self-help groups and voluntary organizations or fee-for-service professional care. In the latter case, the alcoholics could decide themselves whether the treatment is worth their money. The cost of rational professional treatment is not exceedingly high. Attaining abstinence or moderate drinking increases success in the treatment for the possible underlying problems.

172

VII

WHAT AILS THE DOMINANT ALCOHOL POLICY THEORIES

174

The great social experiments by humans on humans - imperialism, communism and prohibition - have brought about much misery, organized crime and corrupted government. Some trends suggest that these monsters are only hibernating, not dead. Calls for stricter alcohol policies echo the slogans of prohibition.

Alcohol intake remains a major issue in many societies. Several interest groups exist and stand in conflict. Because of these long-lasting conflicts, strong emotions escalate and undermine rational policy-making. Temperance, health and welfare organizations tend to magnify the harms of alcohol intake and belittle or renounce the benefits. Producers and sellers may act contrariwise. This has led to fruitless vituperation. We need constructive discussion and open-minded review of the current alcohol policy ideas. In my opinion, the dominant ideas at present are based on shaky premises. Current estimates of the social costs of drinking are unscientific, inflated, and serve only anti-drinking propaganda. High taxes and restricted availability of alcoholic beverages decrease both the consumption and health level of moderate users while having no notable effect on alcoholics. The latter suffer most of the death and disease due to alcohol. Misguided theories uphold ineffectual policies.

175

25 The size of the problem - Inflated figures sell best

Hot air makes the problem inflate nicely.

Estimates on the global burden of alcohol intake have considered that the theoretical minimum-risk exposure is that of no alcohol consumption (Lim et al. 2012). This overestimates the burden because beneficial effects are being neglected. Calculations based on the dose-response estimates of relative risk are biased because published meta-analyses, as Part I has shown, have excluded studies showing a weaker relation between heavy alcohol intake and mortality. Wide variation in the global burden due to alcohol is likely if estimates derived by different methods were compared. In France, comparison of several methods found that the estimated number of deaths varied from 7 % caused by alcohol to 18 % prevented by alcohol (Rey et al. 2010).

Diagnoses with mention of alcohol are considered 100 % due to alcohol. These are called alcohol-specific diagnoses. There are two pitfalls here. First, alcohol-specific diseases also have other risk factors than alcohol. Secondly, every new revision of the International Classification of Diseases (ICD) has more alcohol-specific diagnoses than the previous one. In the 1960's, the ICD-8 included five alcohol-specific diagnoses, the current ICD-10 has 64 items in Finland. The 2010 version of ICD-10 published by WHO seems to include at least 100 three-digit alcohol codes. Some have found about 200 codes where alcohol is a component cause at this level. National modifications of ICD often have five-digit codes which expands the likelihood of harvesting more alcohol-related diseases. The more you label, the more problems that rear their ugly heads.

The problem of alcohol-specific diseases

Making a cause-of-death diagnosis is like looking in a rear-view mirror. You see the outcome and you try to figure out what were the causes of what you see. Seldom only one probable cause emerges. Age correlates with the number and severity of diseases. The more diseases and risk factors that present themselves, the more possible causes that must be considered. This makes selecting one cause as the underlying (main) cause subject to both random error and biases due to diagnostic fashion and moral judgments. How else could we explain the difference between Finland and Ireland. Liver cirrhosis mortality has increased steeply in Finland in step with per capita alcohol intake but no such increase has taken place in Ireland in spite of rising consumption (Sheron et al. 2008). In 2004, per capita alcohol consumption was 12.5 liters in Finland and 14.4 liters in Ireland. Not a big difference. However, age-standardized liver cirrhosis mortality per 100,000 of population was 13.2 in Finland and only 4.4 in Ireland. Moreover, the percentage of alcohol-specific deaths in

177

this category was 87 % in Finland but 53 % in Ireland.

Alcohol-specific diseases are entities with alcohol mentioned in the name of the disease, that is the diagnosis. The terminology is not uniform because sometimes these diagnoses are called alcohol-related or alcohol-attributable diseases (or causes of death). It is hard to find diseases with only a single cause. As to alcohol-specific diseases, alcohol is the cause only in a logical sense, necessary because it is included in the name. Likewise in road traffic accidents, roads are a necessary cause because they also appear in the name. To select only one cause out of many is to fall into the essentialistic trap - the mono-causal view of disease causation. This view is too simplistic. It seems credible only if you refuse to see other factors. For example, if you ask a medical student what is the cause of poliomyelitis, the answer is likely to be the poliovirus. Responding cannot be easier than that because the virus was named after the disease, and the name actually covers not one but three enteroviruses that can cause poliomyelitis under certain conditions. The answer ignores other causal influences relating to genetic susceptibility, bad hygiene, lack of vaccination and low resistance, among others. Several factors together constitute a sufficient train of causation. Infection is a necessary, but not a sufficient, cause of an infectious disease. Humans may carry many kinds of bacteria and viruses without any harm.

To call a disease alcohol-specific is sensible only if the disease can be eradicated by removing risky alcohol intake, just like poliomyelitis by vaccination. The question then is what is risky intake - at least what is the risk level, the risk rhythm and the risky speed of drinking - and what is needed for its elimination. As long as there are no effective and easy way to prevent risky alcohol intake, talk about alcohol as the cause of alcohol-specific diseases does not serve anymore than strident propaganda claims. The scientific value is as great as the swimming trunks of Donald Duck. Alcohol-specific diseases have also other risk factors than alcohol. Genes play a modest role. Genetic variants can be combined to polygenic scores to study their relation to behavioral traits or disease outcomes. The scores can consist of data on thousands of genetic variants and statistical weights in order to improve the strength of the relation. A large study found that polygenic scores had significant, but small associations of self-reported alcohol amount with alcohol-specific deaths and hospital associations. Compared with the group with the lowest scores that with the highest ones had 1.3-1.8-fold risk for death or diagnosis from alcohol-specific diseases (Kiiskinen et al. 2020). Alcohol-specific hospital admissions have been found to be related to living in a deprived area and smoking in addition to alcohol (Gartner et al. 2019). The many risk factors of liver cirrhosis have been mentioned already in the chapter 15 on liver cirrhosis.

Cost of harm estimates – good for indoctrination

Worldwide, the anti-alcohol business loves to estimate the

social costs of alcohol use with the aim to convince politicians and the public that alcohol intake is cost generating and great savings would accrue by doing away with the devil drink. Hidden in the calculations you will find computation errors, logical somersaults, false assumptions based on shaky premises and pious moralism (Mäkelä 2012). Calculations of indirect costs are even more precarious than those for direct ones. The anti-drinking clique argues that politicians want price tags. There is a conflict between the desire to support an anti-drinking partisan program and scientific honesty.

The underlying logic of cost-of-alcohol harm studies

Because some kinds of alcohol use produce harms, related costs can be estimated. Monetary expenditure can be used to argue that population alcohol consumption needs to be decreased. If we accept monetary calculations as the only guide to alcohol policy, then we should also calculate the monetary gains. For example, the immediate public costs of alcohol use have been estimated to be approximately 1.7 billion dollars (1.7 milliard euros) in Finland. But the respective tax income is 2.9 billion dollars, leaving a profit of 1.2 billion dollars. No attention is paid to the savings due to beneficial effects, which would alter the results radically. In Finland in 2010, the annual sales of beverages came to 6.8 billion dollars, including also an estimate of the popular tax-free sales. Judging from the spending habits of the public, the direct benefits seem to be higher.

If monetary gains guide decision-making, then a further profit increase could be realized, for instance, by providing all alcoholics as much as they want of free alcohol. And why? Because this would likely lead to the demise of a large number of alcoholics, therefore eliminating health and social care costs that would otherwise accrue later. Even the hardest drink-haters would reject this economic reasoning if they understood where it would ultimately lead. Fortunately, decisions are based not only on monetary values but also on moral ones.

Every consumer makes his or her own value judgments, either rationally or unconsciously. When these are put together and reported as population averages in survey studies, we find that both positive and negative consequences increase by the amount of alcohol intake and frequency of intoxication. At every intake level the scores of positive consequences are higher than the negative ones except at the highest level where there is no material difference (Leigh 1999; Mäkelä and Mustonen 1988; Nyström 1992). The balance is positive for moderate drinkers.

181

26 Errors in the dominant theory

"It is clear that each society or state must arrive at its own combination of preventive strategies in the light of its historical experience and political composition."
Bruun et al. 1975

In 1842, when Abraham Lincoln (1809 ~ 1865) was addressing the temperance folks in Springfield, Illinois, he famously said that "none seemed to think the injury arose from the use of a bad thing, but from the abuse of a very good thing"(Lincoln 1842). The belief that we are dealing with the use of a bad thing continues to dominate the policy. The dominant dogma claims that it is necessary to reduce the population total alcohol consumption by increasing the price and reducing the availability of the beverages in order to diminish the alcohol-related harms. This is called the total consumption model (Room et al. 2005). The claims were originally presented in a pivotal book entitled *Alcohol Control Policies in Public Health Perspective* (Bruun et al. 1975). The authors of this book, being aware of the weaknesses of their argumentation, made their conclusions with great reservations. If they had known then what is known now, perhaps they would have written otherwise. Nevertheless, the theory is nowadays thought to be as watertight as concrete. In 1994, a book entitled *Alcohol Policy and the Public Good* (Edwards et al. 1994) stated that

"The research established beyond doubt that public health measures of proven effectiveness are available to serve the public good by reducing the widespread costs and pain related to alcohol use. To that end, it is appropriate to deploy responses that influence both the total amount of alcohol consumed by a population and the high risk contexts and drinking behaviors that are so often associated with alcohol-related problems.". But concrete is not watertight in the long run.

The hidden ideology of the total consumption model

How did this model come about? In some countries the anti-alcohol movement achieved its final goal - prohibition, leading then to a dismal failure. It seemed impossible to try it again, despite prohibition's positive influence on liver disease mortality. Politically more feasible was the attempt to try to decrease overall alcohol consumption as much as possible. Scientific support for this policy was sought for, found and marketed. In spite of an emphasis on science, the total consumption model resembles more a tool for a social movement rather than a scientific quest of truth. Robin Room wrote "In many ways Klaus [Mäkelä] and I always remained 1960s student movement radicals studying social change, especially why change is so difficult to achieve. .. So we built research teams as if we were building a social movement and we were determined to figure out social change, asking how

183

governments can get their alcohol policy so wrong, and what needs to be done to get that to change." [12]

Apparently the total alcohol consumption model can be compared to simplified views of classic economics. For example, Jean-Baptiste Say (1767-1832) is known for his claims on the relation between the production and consumption of goods. A popular version of Say's law states that supply creates its own demand. So the better the availability and the lower the price of alcoholic beverages the higher the consumption. An anti-alcohol researcher might have thought that a good way to diminish demand is to decrease the supply of alcoholic beverages by high taxation and austere restriction. This makes sense the views of classic and neoclassic schools of economics are to be believed. Their theories assume that consumers are rational. The *homo economicus* coolly calculates costs and benefits and reacts accordingly to price changes. The school of behavioral economics which includes several Nobel prize winners, has shown that this is simply not true. The total consumption model is not factually supported when all the evidence is examined, and not merely cherry-picked through various studies.

Three major claims were made in *Alcohol Control Policies in Public Health Perspective.* First, in any population,

---

[12]   A book of letters for Robin Room: celebrating fifty years of research and service. No publication date nor place. page 59. Available also at https://dpmp.unsw.edu.au/resource/room [accessed December 19, 2014]

the amount of alcohol consumption will be distributed skewed between the consumers so that a small percentage of drinkers will consume a great amount of alcohol and the large majority will consume smaller amounts. The former were named heavy consumers. Roughly, the 10 % of heavy consumers would drink one half of all alcohol. The higher the average consumption in a population, the higher is the number of heavy consumers. Secondly, the higher the number of heavy consumers, the more are the harms. Consequently, if the number of heavy consumers decreases, the harms will also fall. Thirdly, the decline will be achieved by increasing the price and reducing the availability of beverages. Let us review the evidence.

The skewed distribution

The first claim seems to be true at first sight. Most distributions of alcohol consumption in populations are skewed, and approximate a theoretical statistical model of lognormal distributions that has only one parameter. This is the average. It determines the shape of the curve. The curve has only one hump, not two. This was taken to mean that there is no difference between alcoholics and other consumers. However, one cannot rule out the possibility that the curve was a result of amalgamating distributions of the above two populations (Miller and Agnew 1974). It has long been known that the presence of two distributions is difficult to detect in practice if bimodality is very slight (Harris and Smith 1947). While there

185

may not be a sharp distinction between the long-term amount of alcohol intake between the two groups the rhythm and blood alcohol levels will show more difference, as we saw earlier when alcoholism was discussed. Alcoholics are underrepresented in population surveys that provide the evidence at hand. A small group does not necessarily have any substantial influence on the total population distribution of average alcohol intake reports. In France, after adjustment for underestimation of alcohol intake, the percentage of heaviest consumers increased clearly and the distribution had two humps (Rey et al. 2010).

Surveys inform about what we can see in a population at a specified period or point in time. Lognormal models are fine for this. However, they are not good for predicting what will happen. Change remains unknown. Thus, we cannot know if it is the average alcohol intake that determines the number of heavy consumers or is it the other way around. Maybe it is not the tail that wags the dog.

Heavy drinkers and harm

Secondly, the claim that the higher the number of heavy consumers, the more are the harms. This was based both on cross-sectional, time-series and follow-up data on mortality. Cross-nationally, there were correlations between per capita alcohol consumption and liver cirrhosis mortality. However, the strength of the correlation varied.

As evidence, time-series data on alcohol and liver

cirrhosis in various countries were presented (Bruun et al. 1975). Sometimes the variation was in the same direction, sometimes in a different direction and sometimes there was no clear covariation. Later studies have found similar results (Ramstedt 2001; Norström and Ramstedt 2005). However, time-series studies observe national or other large population group data. These are subject to many potential biases.

First, contrary to data on individuals, we cannot be sure that the alcohol exposure and the outcome reside in the same person when aggregated population data are used. It is not easy to understand why the number of heavily partying young males in a population should correlate with high liver cirrhosis mortality among old women. Secondly, time-series data, say on consecutive calendar years, are not independent observations. Therefore, special statistical time-series models must be employed. These series usually need to be rather long. Close to one hundred observations would be nice. During such long time-periods, societies change in many ways that may bias the relation between the two variables under study - alcohol and harm. The borders and the ethnic composition of the population, principles of statistical data collection and categorization, living habits and risk factor distributions may all change. Thirdly, controlling for other potentially causal factors is often impossible or restricted to only a few ones among all the relevant ones. These are perhaps discussed as weaknesses in the studies but not taken into account when the conclusion is presented to the public.

187

Interpretation of short- and long-term changes is undermined by the practical limitations of the time-series methodology and the plenitude of outcome measures. For example, after the tax cuts in Finland, alcohol-related mortality increased while both cardiovascular and, more importantly, all-cause mortality either decreased or did not change significantly, depending on the age-group under study (Herttua 2011). You can prove almost anything with time-series methods. If you want to support your preconceptions just select the part of the results that supports it.

At the time of the publication of *Alcohol Control Policies in Public Health Perspective* in 1975, not much was known about the higher occurrence of harms among heavy consumers. Therefore, evidence of harms was based on the mortality of alcoholics. Follow-up studies showed that alcoholics, after treatment for this condition, had considerably higher mortality than the population in general, even when age and sex were standardized indirectly. The mistake is that not all of this excess mortality is due to high alcohol intake. Later studies have shown that a great deal of the excess deaths are due to smoking-related causes and poor dental hygiene (Hurt et al. 1996; Poikolainen et al. 2011; Sabbah et al. 2013). Other possible risk factors include poor nutrition, lack of exercise and low social group. Nutritious diet, even when alcohol intake continues, can reverse many health problems in alcoholics (Green 1983). One additional risk indicator is divorce (Poikolainen et al. 2011). The first evidence on the mortality of alcoholics compared with other drinkers came from a cohort of almost 38,000 adults who represented the population of the USA (Dawson 2000a). Many other risk factors were controlled for. These included age, gender, marital status, education, income, smoking, obesity and self-reported poor health. Compared with lifelong abstainers, subjects both with alcoholism (DSM-IV alcohol dependence criteria) and a daily average alcohol intake of four standard drinks (52 g, equaling 2.24 oz.) or more had a 1.65-fold risk of death (95% CI 1.38 - 1.98). There was no material difference in mortality between lifelong abstainers and very heavy drinkers who were not alcoholics, even if the long-term daily average drinking level was approximately equal to that of alcoholics. This agrees well with the estimates of the risk level presented above in Part I. Compared with lifelong abstainers, the relative risk for moderate drinkers (6 - 29 g/day) was 0.86 (95% CI 0.79 - 0.93). Recently, a large Swedish study has found similar results (Lundin et al. 2015). The main risk factor is not heavy intake but heavy intake with alcoholic drinking habits.

What will be achieved by increasing the price and reducing the availability of the beverages?

There is no convincing explanation why the growth of per capita alcohol consumption should necessarily increase the consumption of everybody. A kind of infection mechanism has been suggested. If you drink more, then I will drink more, too.

This may be true in some social situations but not in others. It is not plausible that if I drink more alone, some other people in someplace else will also drink more. Nor is it probable that if you drink less there is an alcoholic who will also drink less. Moreover, it does not seem ethical to demand that moderate drinkers should cut down their intake or abstain, thus increasing their risk of disease, just to ease the way for alcoholics to reduce drinking.

Price and alcohol consumption

Some cross-regional and cross-national studies have found that price increases and reductions of availability can lead to a decrease in alcohol consumption. Some other studies have found the opposite or no change (Mäkelä et al. 2008). Time-series studies typically find that small increases in price are related to even smaller decreases in alcohol consumption. One large meta-analysis found that one per cent increase translates into an average decrease of 0.5 per cent of beer, 0.7 per cent of wine and 0.8 per cent of spirits consumption (Wagenaar et al. 2009). The figures vary by time and place. These are not universal constants. Some effect on alcohol consumption has been observed in some studies but others have not found any effect (Wagenaar et al. 2009, Dumont et al. 2017). Overall, the putative effects are small. Large price increases are likely to be needed to bring about bigger changes. However, such increases may produce unwanted effects that the simple time-series models cannot foresee.

The above pertains to the total population. The more interesting question is: does the decrease affect all consumption groups similarly or are there differences in the outcome. And in fact, a large study on individual changes has shown that price does not significantly affect the alcohol consumption of heavy drinkers while the larger population group of moderate drinkers is sensitive to price changes (Ayyagari et al. 2009). Likewise, time-series studies show that price and tax increases have less effect on heavy drinking than on the drinkers in general. In this case, a one per cent increase was followed by an average decrease of 0.28 in alcohol intake (Wagenaar et al. 2009). This is due to the fact that total alcohol consumption is more strongly associated with the proportions of abstainers and heavy drinkers than that of moderate drinkers in a population (Poikolainen 2017a). Because of their disposition, alcoholics are likely to be more resistant to price increases than heavy drinkers. For alcoholics, booze is almost always worth the price. Examples in the USA and the late Soviet Union, presented below, will show what happens when availability is tightened to the extreme.

Price and health consequences

The pivotal question is what effects on health price increases and other measures aiming to decrease demand of alcohol will have. Population alcohol consumption statistics do not count non-beverage alcohol but intake of such surrogates may have a marked impact on health. In Finland, deaths from

191

alcohol poisoning increased rapidly from one year to another between 1961-1968 although the recorded alcohol sales remained low. The poor alcoholics drank denatured industrial 94 % ethyl alcohol. After liberalization of alcohol laws in 1969 beer came widely available. Sales control was relaxed, and the drunkards were allowed to buy legally available alcoholic beverages. Consequently, recorded alcohol consumption increased considerably but no further increase from alcohol poisoning deaths was noted.

Price and availability do not seem to have much influence on alcohol-related health. A cross-regional study compared states in the USA. Liver cirrhosis mortality correlated clearly with average alcohol consumption per capita, but only if no other factors were taken into account. A multivariate analysis did not show any significant association for liver cirrhosis with alcohol consumption, price level, alcohol availability and tourism. Only urbanization and the percentage of those living alone were significantly related to liver cirrhosis mortality (Colón et al. 1981).

Alcoholics are resistant to price upturns but vulnerable to price decreases under certain conditions. When alcohol tax cuts were made in Finland, a considerable increase was observed in alcohol-specific mortality among those groups in the working-age population who were either unemployed or on a work-disability pension. No such change was seen among those who were employed (Herttua 2010).

It is true that harms may accrue even to people drinking

192

less than alcoholics. This, however, is a poor argument for decreasing the average population consumption. Most harms accrue to those who prefer to drink heavily at a time and aim at intoxication like alcoholics do (Dawson 2000a; Poikolainen et al. 2007). For example, you can see from one follow-up study that 93 % of all alcohol-specific deaths and 96 % of life-years considered to be lost before the age of 65 years due to these deaths occurred among men who reported heavy drinking occasions or had heavy average alcohol intake (Poikolainen et al. 2007).

Disability-adjusted life years (DALYs) are thought to be the most comprehensive measure of health. DALYs are composites of the number of years lost due to ill-health, disability and premature death. One DALY equals one lost year of healthy life. The calculation is complex and contains several assumptions. There are two components. One is the number of potential life years lost due to premature mortality. To get this, one has to decide on an imaginary maximal life span, before which a death is considered to be premature. This span can vary from country to country and be different for men and women. To these lost life years you then add the product of disease duration (from onset to cure or death) multiplied by a disability weight. Weights vary from zero to one. For example, the weight for a severe disease may be 0.8, meaning that 80% of the time with the disease is considered to be time with a disability. The weights have been determined by a small group

193

of experts. Some call them guesstimates.[13]

Alcohol Policy Index is a composite indicator comprising regulations from five policy domains: availability (restrictions to access) of alcohol, drinking context, alcohol prices, alcohol advertising, and motor vehicle driving restrictions. These policies have been sponsored by the World Health Organization (WHO) in the hope of decreasing the adverse effects of alcohol. It is claimed that alcohol-related harms will diminish if the population total alcohol consumption is reduced by increasing the price, lessening availability and controlling the marketing of beverages. In fact, there is evidence that banning or restricting marketing would not decrease alcohol consumption (Siegfried et al. 2014).

I gauged the severity of alcohol control policies by the Alcohol Policy Index. I found that the severity of alcohol policy had no association with the number of alcohol-related DALYs in 30 OECD countries in 2005. Moreover, there no association with alcohol consumption (Poikolainen 2016a). The rate of excise tax on alcoholic beverages was not related to alcohol-related DALYs (25 countries with tax rate data). The findings disagree strongly with the total consumption model. This study has several strengths: data from 30 similar developed OECD countries, a comprehensive outcome

---

[13] DALYs have been criticized for having flawed assumptions and value judgments, failing to give enough emphasis to the poor, low social class, and low treatment potential.

measure, control of confounding built into the risk estimates attributed to alcohol, either derived from studies adjusting for confounding factors or from judgments by the cause-of-death examiners, and high power because R^2 was large and the number of explanatory variables limited (Poikolainen 2017b).

If policy becomes more stringent, moderate drinkers are likely to decrease their drinking. Heavy drinkers and alcoholics are less sensitive to severe control measures. Therefore, strict policies may bring about fewer health benefits to moderate drinkers but make little change in the health of alcoholics. In the worst case, stringent alcohol policies can lead to counterproductive effects, such as illicit trade and moonshining as well as consuming industrial alcohol products that have high toxicity, thus killing more alcoholics.

"Natural experiments" in unnatural conditions

The last form of argument by the proponents of the total consumption model is the so-called natural experiment. In extreme conditions large changes can sometimes be observed. During World War I, strict limitations of alcohol availability took place in Great Britain, Germany and Russia because these countries were in a state of war. The limitations were not applied to the soldiers, however. The French rank-and-file defended Verdun drinking *pinard*, the cheap and rough wine. The Russian soldiers got 100 grams of vodka daily, 200 grams before the attack to raise the offensive spirits. Denmark was not

195

in a state of war but because of grain shortage, large tax increases were enacted. These were followed by big decreases in mortality from alcohol psychosis and poisoning. During World War II, liver cirrhosis mortality decreased sharply in Paris when wine was rationed during the occupation of France. During the Prohibition in the USA in 1920-1933, liver cirrhosis mortality decreased but not sharply. Illegal and sacramental alcohol was widely available. In 1930, the average alcohol consumption was 1.8 gallons, that is 6.8 liters (Leake and Silverman 1966 p. 133). It was commonly said that Prohibition was better than no liquor at all (Okrent 2010). There was more crime on the streets, corruption in politics and organization by the mob.

In the Soviet Union, mortality decreased for the first three years of the glasnost temperance campaign which decreased alcohol availability. Then the backlash kicked in. More moonshine and industrial alcohol, laced with toxic substances, was consumed. Tax income decreased, then the economy went sour. After the breakdown of the workers' paradise, mortality was higher than before the reform (Leon 2011).

Perhaps the most intensive anti-alcohol campaign in the world is going on in North Korea. Production is minuscule and there is no alcohol marketing except one beer advertisement, allowed for patriotic reasons. Despite this, alcohol has been estimated to decrease disability-adjusted life years by 6 %.[14]

---

[14] www.healthmetricsandevaluation.org/gbd/country-

196

The respective proportion in the USA with its large abstinent population is 4.5 % and in France with its liberal alcohol policies slightly less than 6.5 %.

In North Korea, the restrictive alcohol policy results in compensating home brewing. Two pounds of corn yields one quart of brew with 25 % of alcohol, doubling the black market price.[15] Meals are avoided when drinking in order to maximize drunkenness.

The above shows that "natural experiments" are possible in unnatural conditions. Do we desire war, crime or economic breakdown? Would we accept austere and counterproductive reforms under normal conditions? Some anti-alcohol partisans present these conditions as desirable. They won in the USA in the 1920's. Can they win again? Only if we are not alert.

A fresh look at alcohol policy

The anti-alcohol lobby is a strong one. It includes the anti-alcohol academics and ex-temperance societies now masquerading as public health organizations. Many of these are being funded from governmental or EU sources. The lobby has succeeded in marketing their model so well that the WHO now recommends this *one size fits all* policy as a universal solution. This is in stark contrast to the view that each society should arrive at its own combination of preventive strategies in the

profiles -[Accessed July 18th, 2013].

[15]   www.dailynk.com/english/keys/2005/19/03.php   - [Accessed July 18th, 2013].

light of its historical experience and political composition. Who benefits from this domination of the total consumption model? Governments that tax alcoholic beverages, countries that have state alcohol monopolies, bureaucrats that monitor and control the rules and some alcohol researchers who are paid for redundant or biased studies. And who suffer? Moderate drinkers. They are mostly in good health but they are a large group and thus a tempting target for the taxman. This is the paradox.

Alcohol policies need a fresh look. Moderation should be exercised in taxation because it is just one way among many to add to government revenue. Legal restrictions and enforcement are useful in decreasing accidents and violence. However, these measures do not tackle the problems of intoxicating drinking, drunken misbehavior and alcoholism. This is a part of the greater problem of self-control, mental health, aggression and antisocial behavior. Providing suitable work and decent living standards might help as well as education and advising parents in child-rearing. Trials on supporting disadvantaged parents in child-rearing have had some success, although the reviews suggest that the results are meager and more research needs to be done (Barlow et al. 2006; Barlow et al. 2015; Miller et al. 2011).

Crime rates have been decreasing during the past 15 years in many developed and democratic countries. Drinking among youth has decreased in many European countries in the last two decades. Alcohol-attributable mortality has been decreasing in the countries belonging to the WHO European region (Pruckner et al. 2019). Globally, from the year 2000 to 2016, alcohol-attributable deaths have decreased 17.9 per cent and DALYs 14.5 per cent (Shield et al. 2020). Moderation in alcohol intake is spreading in the civilized world without need of a big stick.

REFERENCES

A book of letters for Robin Room: celebrating fifty years of research and service. No publication date nor place. at https://dpmp.unsw.edu.au/resource/room [accessed December 19, 2014].

Ainslie G. *Breakdown of will*, 1st ed. Cambridge, UK: Cambridge University Press, 2001.

Akerstedt T, Connor J, Gray A et al. Predicting road crashes from a mathematical model of alertness regulation - The Sleep/Wake Predictor. *Accid Anal Prev* 2008;40:1480-5.

Alanko T. An overview of techniques and problems in the measurement of alcohol consumption. In: Smart R, Cappell H, Glaser F et al., eds. *Research Advances in Alcohol and Drug Problems, vol. 8.* New York: Plenum, 1984:209-26.

Alexie S. What you pawn I will redeem. In: Furman, Laura, ed. *O. Henry Prize Stories 2005.* Anchor Books, Random House 2005:333-352.

Alha AR. *Blood alcohol and clinical inebriation in Finnish men : a medico-legal study.* Helsinki: Annales Academiae Scientiarum Fennicae. Series A 5, Medica-anthropologica, 26, 1951.

Allen NE, Beral V, Casabonne D et al. Moderate alcohol intake and cancer incidence in women. *J Natl Cancer Inst* 2009;101:296-305.

Amerine MA, Roessler EB. *Wines: their sensory evaluation.* San Francisco: W.H. Freeman, 1976.

Archer T. Effects of exogenous agents on brain development: stress, abuse and therapeutic compounds. *CNS Neurosci Ther* 2011;17:470-89.

Ayyagari P, Deb P, Fletcher J et al.. *Sin taxes: do heterogeneous responses undercut their value?* NBER Working Paper No. 15124, July 2009 (www.nber.org).

Baer DJ, Judd JT, Clevidence BA et al. Moderate alcohol consumption lowers risk factors for cardiovascular disease in postmenopausal women fed a controlled diet. *Am J Clin Nutr* 2002;75:593–599.

Baer HJ, Glynn RJ, Hu FB et al. Risk factors for mortality in the nurses' health study: a competing risks analysis. *Am J Epidemiol* 2011;173:319-29.

Baglietto L, English DR, Hopper JL et al. Average volume of alcohol consumed, type of beverage, drinking pattern and the risk of death from all causes. *Alcohol Alcohol* 2006;41:664-71.

Bagnardi V, Blangiardo M, La Vecchia C et al. A meta-analysis of alcohol drinking and cancer risk. *Br J Cancer* 2001;85:1700-5.

201

Barlow J, Bennett C, Midgley N et al. Parent-infant psychotherapy for improving parental and infant mental health. *Cochrane Database of Systematic Reviews* 2015, Issue 1. Art. No.: CD010534. DOI: 10.1002/14651858.CD010534.pub2

Barlow J, Johnston I, Kendrick D et al. Individual and group-based parenting programmes for the treatment of physical child abuse and neglect. *Cochrane Database of Systematic Reviews* 2006, Issue 3. Art. No.: CD005463. DOI: 10.1002/14651858.CD005463.pub2

Benedict R. *The Chrysanthemum and the sword.* London: Routledge & Kegan Paul 1967.

Bernhoft IM, Behrensdorff I. Effect of lowering the alcohol limit in Denmark. *Accid Anal Prev* 2003;35:515-25.

Berthat H. *Vingt chansons du vin de Bourgogne.* Dijon: Èditions Latitudes-L'Harmattan, 1995.

Beulens JW, van den Berg R, Kok FJ et al. Moderate alcohol consumption and lipoprotein-associated phospholipase A2 activity. *Nutr Metab Cardiovasc Dis* 2008;18:539–544.

Blum RH. On the presence of demons. In: Richard II. Blum & associates. *Society and drugs I: Social and cultural observations.* San Francisco: Jossey-Bass, 1969:323-41.

Bonita JS, Mandarano M, Shuta D, Vinson J. Coffee and cardiovascular disease: in vitro, cellular, animal, and human studies. *Pharmacol Res* 2007;55:187-98.

Bretteville-Jensen A.L. Addiction and discounting. *J Health Econ* 1999;18:393-407.

Brien SE, Ronksley PE, Turner BJ et al. Effect of alcohol consumption on biological markers associated with risk of coronary heart disease: systematic review and meta-analysis of interventional studies. *BMJ* 2011;342:d636. doi: 10.1136/bmj.d636.

Briggs DE, Boulton CA, Brookes PA et al. *Brewing science and practice.* Woodhead Publishing, 2004.

Brinton EA. Effects of ethanol intake on lipoproteins and atherosclerosis. *Curr Opin Lipidol.* 2010;21(4):346–351. doi:10.1097/MOL.0b013e32833c1f41

Brochet F, Dubourdieu D. Wine descriptive language supports cognitive specificity of chemical senses. *Brain and Language* 2001;77:187–196.

Brochet F. The taste of wine in consciousness. *Journal International des Sciences de la Vigne et du Vin*: Special Issue Wine Tasting, 1999:19–22.

Brodsky A, Peele S. Psychosocial benefits of moderate alcohol consumption: alcohol's role in a broader conception of health and well-being. In: Peele S, Grant M, eds. *Alcohol and pleasure: a health perspective.* Philadelphia: Taylor & Francis 1999:187-207.

Bruun K, Edwards G, Lumio M et al. *Alcohol control policies in public health perspective.* Forssa: Finnish Foundation for Alcohol Studies, vol. 25, 1975.

203

Bruun K, Markkanen T. *Onko alkoholismi parannettavissa?* Helsinki: Väkijuomakysymyksen tutkimussäätiön julkaisuja, no 11, 1961.

Casey BJ, Somerville LH, Gotlib IH et al. Behavioral and neural correlates of delay of gratification 40 years later. *Proc Natl Acad Sci USA* 2011;108:1498-5003.

Chick J. Alcohol dependence - an illness with a treatment? *Addiction* 1993;88:1481-92.

Colón I, Cutter HS, Jones WC. Alcohol control policies, alcohol consumption, and alcoholism. *Am J Drug Alcohol Abuse* 1981;8:347-62.

Combs-Orme T, Taylor JR, Robins LN et al. Differential mortality among alcoholics by sample site. *Am J Public Health* 1983;73:900-3.

Corrao G, Lepore AR, Torchio P et al. The effect of drinking coffee and smoking cigarettes on the risk of cirrhosis associated with alcohol consumption. A case-control study. *Eur J Epidemiol* 1994;10:657-64.

Dai J, Mukamal KJ, Krasnow RE et al. Higher usual alcohol consumption was associated with a lower 41-y mortality risk from coronary artery disease in men independent of genetic and common environmental factors: the prospective NHLBI Twin Study. *Am J Clin Nutr* 2015;102:31–9.

Dawson DA, Grant BF, Stinson FS et al. Recovery from DSM-IV alcohol dependence: United States, 2001-2002. *Addiction* 2005;100:281-92.

Dawson DA, Smith SM, Saha TD et al.. Comparative performance of the AUDIT-C in screening for DSM-IV and DSM-5 alcohol use disorders. *Drug Alcohol Depend* 2012;26:384-8.

Dawson DA. Alcohol consumption, alcohol dependence, and all-cause mortality. *Alcohol Clin Exp Res* 2000a;24:72-81. See also Erratum in: *Alcohol Clin Exp Res* 2000;24:395.

Dawson DA. Drinking patterns among individuals with and without DSM-IV alcohol use disorders. *J Stud Alcohol* 2000b;61:111-20.

de la Bedoyere M. *Francis: A Biography of The Saint of Assisi.* Collins 1962.

de Lint J. Alcohol consumption and liver cirrhosis mortality: the Netherlands, 1950-78. *J Stud Alcohol* 1981;42:48-56.

de Saint-Exupéry A. *The little prince.* New York: Reynal & Hitchcock, 1943.

Desapriya EB, Iwase N. Impact of the 1970 legal BAC 0.05 mg % limit legislation on drunk-driver-involved traffic fatalities, accidents, and DWI in Japan. *Subst Use Misuse* 1998;33:2757-88.

Desapriya E, Pike I, Subzwari, S et al. Impact of lowering the legal blood alcohol concentration limit to 0.03 on male, female and teenage drivers involved alcohol-related crashes in Japan. *Int J Injury Control Safety Promotion* 2007;14:181-187.

Di Castelnuovo A, Costanzo S, Bagnardi V et al. Alcohol dosing and total mortality in men and women: an updated meta-analysis of 34 prospective studies. *Arch Intern Med* 2006;166:2437-45.

Dickson Wright C. *Spilling the beans.* London: Hodder & Stoughton, 2007.

Drinking games: How much people drink may matter less than how they drink it. https://www.newyorker.com/magazine/2010/02/15/drinking-games

Duhigg C. *The power of habit: why we do what we do and how to change.* London: William Heinemann, 2012.

Dumont S, Marques-Vidal P, Favrod-Coune T et al. Alcohol policy changes and 22-year trendsin individual alcohol consumption in a Swiss adult population: a 1993-2014 cross-sectional population-based study. *BMJ Open* 2017 ;7:e014828. Doi: 10.1136/bmjopen-2016-014828.

Ebrahim S, Davey Smith G. Mendelian randomization: can genetic epidemiology help redress the failures of observational epidemiology? *Hum Genet* 2008;123:15-33.

Edenberg HJ, McClintick JN. Alcohol Dehydrogenases, Aldehyde Dehydrogenases, and Alcohol Use Disorders: A Critical Review. *Alcohol Clin Exp Res* 2018;42:2281-2297.

Edwards G, Anderson P, Babor TF et al. *Alcohol policy and the public good.* Oxford: Oxford University Press, 1994.

Edwards G, Gross M, Keller M et al. *Alcohol-related disabilities* (WHO Offset Publication No 32). Geneva: World Health Organization, 1977.

Edwards G, Kyle E, Nicholls P et al. Alcoholism and correlates of mortality. Implications for epidemiology. *J Stud Alcohol* 1978;39:1607-17.

Ellison GD, Potthoff AD. Social models of drinking behavior in animals. The importance of individual differences. *Recent Dev Alcohol* 1984;2:17-36.

Epictetus. *The Enchiridion.* New york: The Liberal Arts Press 1948. XLVII.

Falgreen Eriksen H, Mortensen E, Kilburn T et al. The effects of low to moderate prenatal alcohol exposure in early pregnancy on IQ in 5-year-old children. *BJOG* 2012;119:1191-200.

Fingarette H. *Heavy drinking: The myth of alcoholism as a disease.* Berkeley, California: University of California Press, 1988.

Flensborg-Madsen T, Knop J, Mortensen EL et al. Amount of alcohol consumption and risk of developing alcoholism in men and women. *Alcohol Alcohol* 2007;42(5):442-7.

Friesema IHM, Zwietering PJ, Veenstra MY et al. Alcohol intake and cardiovascular disease and mortality: The role of pre-existing disease. *J Epid Community Health* 2007; 61:441–446.

Frisher M, Mendonça M, Shelton N et al. Is alcohol

consumption in older adults associated with poor self-rated health? Cross-sectional and longitudinal analyses from the English Longitudinal Study of Ageing. *BMC Public Health* 2015;15:703.

Fuchs CS, Stampfer MJ, Colditz GA et al. Alcohol consumption and mortality among women. *N Engl J Med* 1995;332:1245-50.

Gartner A, Trefan L, Moore S et al. Drinking beer, wine or spirits – does it matter for inequalities in alcohol-related hospital admission? A record-linked longitudinal study in Wales. *BMC Public Health* 2019;19:1651. https://doi.org/10.1186/s12889-019-8015-3.

Gémes K, Moeller J, Engström K et al. Alcohol consumption trajectories and self-rated health: findings from the Stockholm Public Health Cohort. *BMJ Open* 2019;9:e028878. doi: 10.1136/bmjopen-2018-028878.

Gepner Y, Golan R, Harman-Boehm I et al. Effects of Initiating Moderate Alcohol Intake on Cardiometabolic Risk in Adults With Type 2 Diabetes: A 2-Year Randomized, Controlled Trial. *Ann Intern Med* 2015;163:569-79.

Giere RN. *Scientific perspectivism*. Chicago and London: Chicago University Press, 2006.

Gmel G, Gutjahr E, Rehm J. How stable is the risk curve between alcohol and all-cause mortality and what factors influence the shape? A precision-weighted hierarchical meta-analysis. *Eur J Epidemiol* 2003;18:631-42.

Golden J. *Message in the bottle: the making of fetal alcohol syndrome*. Cambridge, Mass.: Harvard University Press, 2005.

Goode J. Experiencing wine, why critics mess up (some of the time). In: Alhoff R. ed. *Wine & Philosophy*. Blackwell, 2008:137-153.

Gordon AJ, Maisto SA, McNeil M, Kraemer KL, Conigliaro RL, Kelley ME, Conigliaro J. Three questions can detect hazardous drinkers. *J Fam Pract* 2001;50:313-20.

Green PH. Alcohol, nutrition and malabsorption. *Clin Gastroenterol* 1983;12:563-74.

Greenland S, Poole C. Living with P-values: Resurrecting a Bayesian perspective. *Epidemiology* 2013;24:62-8.

Grønbæk M, Deis A, Sørensen TIA et al. Mortality associated with moderate intakes of wine, beer, or spirits. *BMJ* 1995;310:1165-9.

Haggard HW, Greenberg LA, Carroll RP. Studies in the absorption, distribution and elimination of alcohol:VIII. the diuresis from alcohol and its influence on the elimination of alcohol in the urine. *J Pharmacol Exp Ther*1941;171:349-357.

Hämäläinen MD, Zetterström A, Winkvist M et al. Breathalyser-Based eHealth Data Suggest That Self-Reporting of Abstinence Is a Poor Outcome Measure for Alcohol Use Disorder Clinical Trials. *Alcohol Alcohol* 2020; agaa004. doi: 10.1093/alcalc/agaa004.

209

Harris H, Smith CAB. The sib-sib age of onset correlation among individuals suffering from a hereditary syndrome produced by more than one gene. *Ann Eugenics* 1947;14:309-18.

Hasin DS, Stinson FS, Ogburn E et al. Prevalence, correlates, disability, and comorbidity of DSM-IV alcohol abuse and dependence in the United States: results from the National Epidemiologic Survey on Alcohol and Related Conditions. *Arch Gen Psychiatry* 2007;64:830-42.

Henderson J, Gray R, Brocklehurst P. Systematic review of effects of low-moderate prenatal alcohol exposure on pregnancy outcome. *BJOG* 2007;114:243-52.

Herttua K. *The effects of the 2004 reduction in the price of alcohol on alcohol-related harm in Finland : A natural experiment based on register data.* Helsinki: Finnish Yearbook of Population Research, 2010.

Herttua K, Mäkelä P, Martikainen P. An evaluation of the impact of a large reduction in alcohol prices on alcohol-related and all-cause mortality: time series analysis of a population-based natural experiment. *Int J Epidemiol* 2011;40:441-54.

Heyman B. The social construction of health risks. In: Heyman B, Shaw M, Alaszewski A, Titterton M. *Risk, safety, and clinical practice.* Oxford: Oxford University Press, 2010.

Heyman GM. *Addiction: a disorder of choice.* Cambridge, Massachusetts: Harvard University Press, 2009.

Higdon JV, Frei B. Coffee and health: a review of recent human research. *Crit Rev Food Sci Nutr* 2006;46:101-23.

Hill AB. The environment and disease: association or causation? *Proc Roy Soc Med* 1965;58:295-300.

Hines LM, Stampfer MJ, Ma J et Genetic variation in alcohol dehydrogenase and the beneficial effect of moderate alcohol consumption on myocardial infarction. *N Engl J Med* 2001;344:549-55.

Holgate JY, Garcia H, Chatterjee S et al. Social and environmental enrichment has different effects on ethanol and sucrose consumption in mice. *Brain Behav* 2017;7:e00767. doi:10.1002/brb3.767

Holmes MV, Dale CE, Zuccolo L et al. Association between alcohol and cardiovascular disease: Mendelian randomisation analysis based on individual participant data. *BMJ* 2014;349:g4164.

Holton R. How is strength of will possible? In: Stroud S, Tappolet C, eds. *Weakness of will and practical irrationality.* Oxford: Clarendon Press, 2007:39-67.

Hume D. Of the standard of taste. In: *Essays, moral, political, and literary.* I.XXIII.18. http://www.econlib.org/library/LFBooks/Hume/hmMPL. html

Hume R, Weyers E. Relationship between total body water and surface area in normal and obese subjects. J *Clin Pathol* 1971;24:234-8.

211

Hurst PM, Harte D, Frith WJ. The Grand Rapids dip revisited. *Accid Anal Prev* 1994;26:647-54.

Hurt RD, Offord KP, Croghan IT et al. Mortality following inpatient addictions treatment: role of tobacco use in a community-based cohort. *JAMA* 1996;275:1097-103.

Huxley RR, Neil HA. The relation between dietary flavonol intake and coronary heart disease mortality: a meta-analysis of prospective cohort studies. *Eur J Clin Nutr* 2003;57:904-8.

Islami F, Pourshams A, Nasrollahzadeh D et al. Tea drinking habits and oesophageal cancer in a high risk area in northern Iran: population based case-control study. *BMJ* 2009;338:b929.

Jayasekara H, MacInnis RJ, Hodge AM et al. Alcohol consumption for different periods in life, intake pattern over time and all-cause mortality. *J Public Health* 2015;37:625-33.

Jonas DE, Garbutt JC, Amick HR et al. Behavioral counseling after screening for alcohol misuse in primary Care: A systematic review and meta-analysis for the U.S. Preventive Services Task Force. *Ann Intern Med* 2012;157:645-54.

Jones AW, Andersson L. Comparison of ethanol concentrations in venous blood and end-expired breath during a controlled drinking study. *Forensic Sci Int* 2003;132:18-25.

Jones AW. Interindividual variations in the disposition and metabolism of ethanol in healthy men. *Alcohol* 1984;1:385-91.

Kalant H. Effects of food and body composition on blood alcohol levels. In: Preedy VR, Watson RR, eds. *Comprehensive Handbook of Alcohol Related Pathology, Volume 1.* Elsevier, 2005:87-101.

Kalant H. What neurobiology cannot tell us about addiction. *Addiction* 2010;105:780-9.

Kalis A, Mojzisch A, Schweizer TS et al. Weakness of will, akrasia, and the neuropsychiatry of decision making: an interdisciplinary perspective. *Cogn Affect Behav Neurosci* 2008;8:402-17.

Kaminski M, Rumeau C, Schwartz D. Alcohol consumption in pregnant women and the outcome of pregnancy. *Alcohol Clin Exp Res* 1978;2:155-63.

Kamper-Jørgensen M, Grønbaek M, Tolstrup J et al. Alcohol and cirrhosis: dose--response or threshold effect? *J Hepatol* 2004;41:25-30.

Kaner EFS, Beyer FR, Muirhead C et al. Effectiveness of brief alcohol interventions in primary care populations. *Cochrane Database of Systematic Reviews* 2018, Issue 2. Art. No.: CD004148. DOI: 10.1002/14651858.CD004148.pub4.

Kelly YJ, Sacker A, Gray R et al. Light drinking in pregnancy, a risk for behavioural problems and cognitive deficits at 3 years of age? *Int J Epidemiol* 2009;38:129-40.

Kelly Y, Iacovou M, Quigley MA et al. Light drinking versus abstinence in regnancy-behavioural and cognitive outcomes in 7-year-old children: a longitudinal cohort study. *BJOG* 2013;120:1340-7.

Kelly YJ, Sacker A, Gray R et al. Light drinking during pregnancy: still no increased risk for socioemotional difficulties or cognitive deficits at 5 years of age? *J Epidemiol Community Health* 2012;66:41-8.

Kiiskinen T, Mars NJ, Palviainen T et al. Genomic prediction of alcohol-related morbidity and mortality. *Transl Psychiatry* 2020;23 https://doi.org/10.1038/s41398-019-0676-2.

Klatsky AL, Armstrong MA. Alcohol, smoking, coffee, and cirrhosis. *Am J Epidemiol* 1992;136:1248-57.

Klatsky AL, Armstrong MA. Alcoholic beverage choice and risk of coronary artery disease mortality: do red wine drinkers fare best? *Am J Cardiol* 1993;71:467-9.

Kleemola P, Jousilahti P, Pietinen P et al. Coffee consumption and the risk of coronary heart disease and death. *Arch Intern Med* 2000;160:3393-400.

Klosse P. *The concept of flavor styles to classify flavors.* Hoog Soeren: Academie voor Gastronomie, 2004.

Knibbe RA, Bloomfield K. Alcohol consumption estimates in surveys in Europe: Comparability and sensitivity for gender differences. *Subst Abus* 2001;22:23-38.

Kunutsor SK. Gamma-glutamyltransferase-friend or foe within? *Liver Int* 2016;36:1723-1734.

Laramée P, Leonard S, Buchanan-Hughes A et al. Risk of All-Cause Mortality in Alcohol-Dependent Individuals: A Systematic Literature Review and Meta-Analysis. *EBioMedicine* 2015;2:1394-404.

Larroque B, Kaminski M, Dehaene P et al. Moderate prenatal alcohol exposure and psychomotor development at preschool age. *Am J Public Health* 1995;85:1654-61.

Larroque B, Kaminski M. Prenatal alcohol exposure and development at preschool age: main results of a French study. *Alcohol Clin Exp Res* 1998:22:998-1040.

Leake CD, Silverman M. *Alcoholic beverages in clinical medicine*. Cleveland: The World Publishing Company by special arrangement with Year Book Medical Publishers, Inc., 1966.

Leigh B. Thinking, feeling, and drinking: alcohol expectancies and alcohol use. In: Peele S, Grant M, eds. *Alcohol and pleasure: a health perspective.* Philadelphia: Taylor & Francis 1999:215-231.

Lelbach WK. Cirrhosis in the alcoholic and its relation to volume of alcohol abuse. *Ann NY Acad Sci* 1975;252:85-105.

Lemoine P, Harousseau H, Borteyru JP et al. Les enfants de parents alcooliques: anomalies observées. A propos de 127 cas. *Ouest Médical* 1968;21:476–482.

Leon DA. Trends in European life expectancy: a salutary view. *Int J Epidemiol* 2011;40:271-7.

Li Y, Schoufour J, Wang DD et al. Healthy lifestyle and life expectancy free of cancer, cardiovascular disease, and type 2 diabetes: prospective cohort study. *BMJ* 2020;368:l6669. doi: 10.1136/bmj.l6669.

Lieber CS, DeCarli L, Rubin E. Sequential production of fatty liver, hepatitis, and cirrhosis in sub-human primates fed ethanol with adequate diets. *Proc Natl Acad Sci USA* 1975;72:437-41.

Lim SS, Vos T, Flaxman AD et al. A comparative risk assessment of burden of disease and injury attributable to 67 risk factors and risk factor clusters in 21 regions, 1990-2010: a systematic analysis for the Global Burden of Disease Study 2010. *Lancet* 2012;380:2224-60.

Lincoln, Abraham. *Temperance address, Springfield, Illinois, February 22, 1842.* http://www.abrahamlincolnonline.org/lincoln/speeches/temperance.htm (Accessed March 23, 2013).

Liskow BI, Powell BJ, Penick EC et al. Mortality in male alcoholics after ten to fourteen years. *J Stud Alcohol* 2000;61:853-61.

Liu B, Balkwill A, Roddam A et al. Separate and joint effects of alcohol and smoking on the risks of cirrhosis and gallbladder disease in middle-aged women. *Am J Epidemiol* 2009;169:153-60.

Loomis, TA. *Essentials of toxicology*, 2nd ed. Philadelphia: Lea & Febiger 1974.

Lundin A, Mortensen LH, Halldin J et al. The Relationship of Alcoholism and Alcohol Consumption to All-Cause Mortality in Forty-One-Year Follow-up of the Swedish REBUS Sample. *J Stud Alcohol Drugs* 2915;76:544-51.

Makarechian N, Agro K, Devlin J et al. Association between moderate alcohol consumption during pregnancy and spontaneous abortion, stillbirth and premature birth: a meta-analysis. *Can J Clin Pharmacol* 1998;5:169–76.

Mäkelä K, Mustonen H. Positive and negative experiences related to drinking as a function of annual alcohol intake. *Br J Addict* 1988;83:403-8.

Mäkelä K. Cost-of-alcohol studies as a research programme. *Nordic Studies on Alcohol and Drugs* 2012;29:321-43.

Mäkelä P, Bloomfield K, Gustafsson NK et al. Changes in volume of drinking after changes in alcohol taxes and travellers' allowances: results from a panel study. *Addiction* 2008;103:181-91.

Mann RE, Macdonald S, Stoduto LG et al. The effects of introducing or lowering legal per se blood alcohol limits for driving: aninte rnational review. *Accid Anal Prev* 2001;33:569-83.

May PA, Gossage JP, Marais AS et al. Maternal risk factors for fetal alcohol syndrome and partial fetal alcohol syndrome in South Africa: a third study. *Alcohol Clin Exp Res* 2008;32:738-53.

McElduff P, Dobson A. How much alcohol and how often? Population based case-control study of alcohol consumption and risk of a major coronary event. *BMJ* 1997;314:1159-64.

Mendelson JH, La Dou J. Experimentally induced chronic intoxication and withdrawal in alcoholics. Part 2. Psychophysiological findings. *Q J Stud Alcohol* 1964;suppl. 2:14-39.

Miller GH, Agnew N. The Ledermann model of alcohol consumption: description, implications and assessment. *Q J Stud Alcohol* 1974;35:877-98.

Miller S, Maguire LK, Macdonald G. Home-based child development interventions for preschool children from socially disadvantaged families. *Cochrane Database of Systematic Reviews* 2011, Issue 12. Art. No.: CD008131. DOI: 10.1002/14651858.CD008131.pub2

Millwood IY, Walters RG, Mei XW et al. Conventional and genetic evidence on alcohol and vascular disease aetiology: a prospective study of 500 000 men and women in China. *Lancet* 2019;393:1831-1842.

Minozzi S, Saulle R, Rösner S. Baclofen for alcohol use disorder. *Cochrane Database of Systematic Reviews* 2018, Issue 11. Art. No.: CD012557. DOI: 10.1002/14651858.CD012557.pub2.

Morean ME, Corbin WR, Fromme K. Age of first use and delay to first intoxication in relation to trajectories of heavy drinking and alcohol-related problems during emerging adulthood. *Alcohol Clin Exp Res* 2012;36:1991-9.

Morrot G, Brochet F, Dubourdieu D. The color of odors. *Brain and Language* 2001;79:309-320.

Newcomb PA, Kampman E, Trentham-Dietz A et al. Alcohol consumption before and after breast cancer diagnosis: associations with survival from breast cancer, cardiovascular disease, and other causes. *J Clin Oncol* 2013; 31:1939-46.

Norberg A, Jones AW, Hahn RG et al. Role of variability in explaining ethanol pharmacokinetics: research and forensic applications. *Clin Pharmacokinet* 2003;42:1-31.

Norström T, Ramstedt M. Mortality and population drinking: a review of the literature. *Drug Alcohol Rev* 2005;24:537-47.

Nyström M. Positive and negative consequences of alcohol drinking among young university students in Finland. *Br J Addict* 1992;87:715-22.

O'Leary CM, Bower C. Guidelines for pregnancy: What's an acceptable risk, and how is the evidence (finally) shaping up? *Drug Alcohol Rev* 2012;31:170–183.

O'Leary CM, Nassar N, Kurinczuk JJ et al. The effect of maternal alcohol consumption on fetal growth and preterm birth. *BJOG* 2009;116:390–400.

O'Leary CM, Nassar N, Zubrick SR et al. Evidence of a complex association between dose, pattern, and timing of prenatal alcohol exposure and child behavior problems. *Addiction* 2010;105:74–86.

Okrent D. *Last call: the rise and fall of Prohibition.* Kindle edition. Scribner, 2010.

Okwuosa TM, Klein O, Chan C et al. Long-term change in alcohol-consumption status and variations in fibrinogen levels: the coronary artery risk development in young adults (CARDIA) study. *BMJ Open* 2013;3(7). doi:pii: e002944. 10.1136/bmjopen-2013-002944.

Oppenheimer GM, Bayer R. Is Moderate Drinking Protective Against Heart Disease? The Science, Politics and History of a Public Health Conundrum. *The Milbank Quarterly* 2019; 5 December doi:10.1111/1468-0009.12437

Orford J, Edwards G. *Alcoholism: a comparison of treatment and advice, with a study of the influence of marriage.* Oxford: Oxford University Press, 1977.

Patra J, Bakker R, Irving H et al. Dose–response relationship between alcohol consumption before and during pregnancy and the risks of low birthweight, preterm birth and small for gestational age (SGA)—a systematic review and meta-analyses. *BJOG* 2011;118:411–1421.

Peacock A, Martin FH, Carr A. Energy drink ingredients. Contribution of caffeine and taurine to performance outcomes. *Appetite* 2013;64:1-4.

Pearl R. *Alcohol and longevity.* New York: Alfred A. Knopf, 1926.

Peele S. *Addiction-proof your child*. New York: Three Rivers Press, 2007.

Peynaud E. *The taste of wine*. London: Macdonald Orbis, 1987.

Piccinelli M, Tessari E, Bortolomasi M et al. Efficacy of the alcohol use disorders identification test as a screening tool for hazardous alcohol intake and related disorders in primary care: a validity study. *BMJ* 1997;314:420-4.

Plato. *Republic*. 380 BC. Translated by Benjamin Jowett. The Project Gutenberg EBook of Plato's Republic. May 22, 2008 [EBook #150]

Poikolainen K. *Alcohol poisoning mortality in four Nordic countries*. Helsinki: Finnish Foundation for Alcohol Studies, Vol. 28, 1977.

Poikolainen K, Kärkkäinen P, Pikkarainen J. Correlations between biological markers and alcohol intake as measured by diary and questionnaire in men. *J Stud Alcohol* 1985;46:383-387.

Poikolainen K, Vartiainen E. Wine and good subjective health. *Am J Epidemiol* 1999;150:47-50.

Poikolainen K. Antecedents of substance use in adolescence. *Curr Opin Psychiatry* 2002;15:241-245.

Poikolainen K. Predictors of alcohol consumption. In: Preedy V, Watson RR, eds. . *Comprehensive Handbook of Alcohol Related Pathology, Volume 1*. Amsterdam, the Netherlands: Elsevier, 2005:49-58.

221

Poikolainen K, Vahtera J, Virtanen M et al. Alcohol and coronary heart disease risk - is there an unknown confounder? *Addiction* 2005;100:1150-1157.

Poikolainen K, Paljärvi T, Mäkelä P. Alcohol and the preventive paradox: serious harms and drinking pattern. *Addiction* 2007;102:571-8.

Poikolainen K. The magic to make the "preventive effect" of alcohol disappear and reappear. *Addiction* 2008;103:1905.

Poikolainen K. Heavy alcohol intake episodes: determinants and interventions. In: de Witte P, ed. *New frontiers in alcohol and health.* Louvain, Belgique: Presses Universitaires de Louvain, 2010:21-40.

Poikolainen K, Paljärvi T, Mäkelä P. Risk factors for alcohol-specific hospitalizations and deaths: prospective cohort study. *Alcohol Alcohol* 2011;46:342-8.

Poikolainen K. The Weakness of Stern Alcohol Control Policies. *Alcohol Alcohol* 2016a;51:93-97.

Poikolainen K. Healthy Former Drinkers Have Higher Mortality Than Light Drinkers. *Alcohol Alcohol* 2016b;51:772-773.

Poikolainen K. Does the Tail Wag the Dog? Abstainers, Alcohol Dependence, Heavy Episodic Drinkers and Total Alcohol Consumption. *Alcohol Alcohol* 2017a;52:80-83.

Poikolainen K. A note on the statistical power of regression analysis. *Alcohol Alcohol* 2017b;52:625

Polygenis D, Wharton S, Malmberg C et al. Moderate alcohol consumption during pregnancy and the incidence of fetal malformations: a meta-analysis. *Neurotoxicol Teratol* 1998;20:61-67.

Pruckner N, Hinterbuchinger B, Fellinger M et al. Alcohol-Related Mortality in the WHO European Region: Sex-Specific Trends and Predictions. *Alcohol Alcohol* 2019;54:593-598.

Public health in England: from nudge to nag. *Lancet* 2012;379:194.

Qiu L, Sautter J, Gu D. Associations between frequency of tea consumption and health and mortality: evidence from old Chinese. *Br J Nutr* 2012;108:1686-97.

Ramstedt M. Per capita alcohol consumption and liver cirrhosis mortality in 14 European countries. *Addiction* 2001;96 Suppl 1:S19-33.

Rey G, Boniol M, Jougla E. Estimating the number of alcohol-attributable deaths: methodological issues and illustration with French data for 2006. *Addiction* 2010;105:1018-29.

Richette P, Bardin T. Gout. *Lancet* 2010;375:318-28.

Ried K, Sullivan TR, Fakler P et al. Effect of cocoa on blood pressure. *Cochrane Database of Systematic Reviews* 2012, Issue 8. Art. No.:CD008893. DOI:10.1002/14651858.CD008893.pub2.

Rimm EB, Klatsky A, Grobbee D et al. Review of moderate alcohol consumption and reduced risk of coronary heart disease: is the effect due to beer, wine, or spirits? *BMJ* 1996;312:731-736.

Rimm EB, Williams P, Fosher K et al. Moderate alcohol intake and lower risk of coronary heart disease: meta-analysis of effects on lipids and haemostatic factors. *BMJ* 1999;319:1523-8.

Rimm EB, Williams P, Fosher K et al. Moderate alcohol intake and lower risk of coronary heart disease: meta-analysis of effects on lipids and haemostatic factors. *BMJ* 1999;319:1523-8.

Rintala J, Jaatinen P, Lu W et al. Effects of lifelong ethanol consumption on cerebellar layer volumes in AA and ANA rats. *Alcohol Clin Exp Res* 1997;21:311-7.

Rintala J, Jaatinen P, Wei L et al. Lifelong ethanol consumption and loss of locus coeruleus neurons in AA and ANA rats. *Alcohol* 1998;16:243-8.

Rodrigo R, Miranda A, Vergara L. Modulation of endogenous antioxidant system by wine polyphenols in human disease. *Clin Chim Acta* 2011;412:410-24.

Rolls E. Willed action, free will, and the stochastic neurodynamics of decision-making. *Front Integr Neurosci* 2012;6:68. doi: 10.3389/fnint.2012.00068

Ronksley PE, Brien SE, Turner BJ et al. Association of alcohol consumption with selected cardiovascular disease outcomes: a systematic review and meta-analysis. *BMJ* 2011;342:d671.

Room R, Babor T, Rehm J. Alcohol and public health. *Lancet* 2005;365:519-30.

Rose S. *Lifelines: life beyond the gene.* London: Vintage, 2005.

Rösner S, Hackl-Herrwerth A, Leucht S et al. Acamprosate for alcohol dependence. *Cochrane Database of Systematic Reviews* 2010a, Issue 9. Art. No.: CD004332. DOI: 10.1002/14651858.CD004332.pub2.

Rösner S, Hackl-Herrwerth A, Leucht S et al. Opioid antagonists for alcohol dependence. *Cochrane Database of Systematic Reviews* 2010b, Issue 12. Art. No.: CD001867. DOI: 10.1002/14651858.CD001867.pub3.

Rossow I, Kuntsche E. Early onset of drinking and risk of heavy drinking in young adulthood - a 13-year prospective study. *Alcohol Clin Exp Res* 2013;37:Suppl 1:E297-304.

Rossow I, Mäkelä P, Kerr W. The collectivity of changes in alcohol consumption revisited. *Addiction* 2014;109:1447-55.

Ruidavets JB, Ducimetière P, Evans A et al. Patterns of alcohol consumption and ischaemic heart disease in culturally divergent countries: the Prospective Epidemiological Study of Myocardial Infarction (PRIME). *BMJ* 2010;341:c6077.

Sabbah W, Mortensen LH, Sheiham A et al. Oral health as a risk factor for mortality in middle-aged men: the role of socioeconomic position and health behaviours. *J Epidemiol Community Health* 2013;67:392-7.

225

Sarviharju M, Riikonen, J, Jaatinen P et al. Survival of AA and ANA rats during lifelong ethanol exposure. *Alcohol Clin Exp Res* 2004;28:93-97.

Saunders JB, Aasland OG, Babor TF et al. Development of the Alcohol Use Disorders Identification Test (AUDIT): WHO Collaborative Project on Early Detection of Persons with Harmful Alcohol Consumption II. *Addiction* 1993;88:791-804.

SBU. *Behandling av alkohol- och narkotikaproblem. En evidensbaserad kunskapssammanställning.* Statens beredning för medicinsk utvärdering, rapport nr 156. Stockholm, 2001. Also available at http://www.sbu.se.

Schmidt W, De Lint J. Social class and the mortality of clinically treated alcoholics. *Br J Addict Alcohol Other Drugs* 1970;64:327-31.

Schmidt W, Popham RE, Israel Y. Dose-specific effects of alcohol on the lifespan of mice and the possible relevance to man. *Br J Addict* 1987;82:775-788.

Schomerus G, Lucht M, Holzinger A et al. The stigma of alcohol dependence compared with other mental disorders: a review of population studies. *Alcohol Alcohol* 2011;46:105-12.

Seneca, L Annaeus Minor. *Moral essays: in three volumes.* London: Heinemann, The Loeb Classical Library, 1964.

Sesso HD, Stampfer MJ, Rosner B et al. Seven-year changes in alcohol consumption and subsequent risk of cardiovascular disease in men. *Arch Intern Med* 2000;160:2605-12.

Sheron N, Olsen N, Gilmore I. An evidence-based alcohol policy. *Gut* 2008;57:1341-4.

Shield K, Manthey J, Rylett M et al. National, regional, and global burdens of disease from 2000 to 2016 attributable to alcohol use: a comparative risk assessment study. *Lancet Public Health* 2020;5:e51-61.

Siegfried N, Pienaar DC, Ataguba JE et al. Restricting or banning alcohol advertising to reduce alcohol consumption in adults and adolescents. *Cochrane Database of Systematic Reviews* 2014, Issue 11. Art. No.: CD010704. DOI: 10.1002/14651858.CD010704.pub2.

Simpson RF, Carol Hermon C, Liu B et al. Alcohol drinking patterns and liver cirrhosis risk: analysis of the prospective UK Million Women Study. *Lancet Public Health*.2019;4:e41-e48.

Slovic P, Fischhoff B, Lichtenstein S. Perceived risk: psychological factors and social implications. *Proc R Soc (London) A* 1981;376:17-34.

Slovic P. Perception of risk. *Science* 1987;236:280-5.

Smith A, Kendrick A, Maben A. Use and effects of food and drinks in relation to daily rhythms of mood and cognitive performance. Effects of caffeine, lunch and alcohol on human performance, mood and cardiovascular function. *Proc Nutr Soc* 1992;51:325-33.

Sood B, Delaney-Black V, Covington C et al. Prenatal alcohol exposure and childhood behavior at age 6 to 7 years: I. dose-response effect. *Pediatrics* 2001;108:E34.

Sørensen TIA. Alcohol and liver injury: dose-related or permissive effect? *Br J Addict* 1989;84:581-589.

Stockwell T, Zhao J, Panwar S et al. Do "Moderate" Drinkers Have Reduced Mortality Risk? A Systematic Review and Meta-Analysis of Alcohol Consumption and All-Cause Mortality. *J Stud Alcohol Drugs* 2016;77:185-98.

Stockwell T. *A review of research into the impacts of alcohol warning labels on attitudes and behaviour.* Centre for Addictions Research of BC, British Columbia, Canada 2006.

Strandberg TE, Strandberg AY, Salomaa VV et al. Alcoholic beverage preference, 29-year mortality, and quality of life in men in old age. *J Gerontol A Biol Sci Med Sci* 2007;313:1362-6.

Streissguth AP, Bookstein FL, Barr HM et al. Risk factors for adverse life outcomes in fetal alcohol syndrome and fetal alcohol effects. *J Dev Behav Pediatr* 2004;25:228-38.

Suter PM, Jéquier E, Schutz Y. Effect of ethanol on energy expenditure. *Am J Physiol* 1994;266:R1204-R1212.

Tabara Y, Ueshima H, Takashima N et al. Mendelian randomization analysis in three Japanese populations supports a causal role of alcohol consumption in lowering low-density lipid cholesterol levels and particle numbers. *Atherosclerosis* 2016;254:242-248.

Testa M, Quigley BM, Eiden RD. The effects of prenatal alcohol exposure on infant mental development: a meta-analytical review. *Alcohol Alcohol* 2003;38:295-304.

The Lancet, editorial. Alcohol and the fetus - is zero the only option? *Lancet* 1983;1:682-683.

Thun MJ, Peto R, Lopez AD et al. Alcohol consumption and mortality among middle-aged and elderly U.S. citizens. *N Engl J Med* 1997;337:1705-14.

Tjønneland A, Grønbæk M, Stripp C et al. Wine intake and diet in a random sample of 48763 Danish men and women. *Am J Clin Nutr* 1999;69:49-54.

Uhl A. Absurditäten in der Suchtforschung. *Wiener Zeitschrift für Suchtforschung* 2009;32:19-39.

Ullmann-Margalit E. Big decisions: opting, converting, drifting. In: O'Hear A., ed. *Political philosophy.* Cambridge, UK: Cambridge University Press, 2006:157-72.

Unreliable research, *The Economist*, October 19 - 25, 2013:21-24.

Urgert R, Meyboom S, Kuilman M et al. Comparison of effect of cafetière and filtered coffee on serum concentrations of liver aminotransferases and lipids: six month randomised controlled trial. *BMJ* 1996;313:1362-6.

van der Gaag MS, Sierksma A, Schaafsma G et al. Moderate alcohol consumption and changes in postprandial lipoproteins of premenopausal and postmenopausal women: a diet-controlled, randomized intervention study. *J Womens Health Gend Based Med* 2000;9:607–616.

Wagenaar AC, Salois MJ, Komro KA. Effects of beverage alcohol price and tax levels on drinking: a meta-analysis of 1003 estimates from 112 studies. *Addiction* 2009;104:179-90.

Wakabayashi I. History of antihypertensive therapy influences the relationships of alcohol with blood pressure and pulse pressure in older men. *Am J Hypertens* 2010;23:633-8. doi: 10.1038/ajh.2010.52.

Wang C, Xue H, Wang Q et al. Effect of drinking on all-cause mortality in women compared with men: a meta-analysis. *J Womens Health* 2014;23:373-81.

Wannamethee SG, Shaper AG. Type of alcoholic drink and risk of major coronary heart disease events and all-cause mortality. *Am J Public Health* 1999;89:685-690.

Warburton DM. Pleasure for health. In: Peele S, Grant M, eds. *Alcohol and pleasure: a health perspective.* Philadelphia: Taylor & Francis 1999:11-23.

Warner LA, White HR. Longitudinal effects of age at onset and first drinking situations on problem drinking. *Subst Use Misuse* 2003;38:1983-2016.

Watson PE, Watson ID, Batt RD. Prediction of blood alcohol concentrations in human subjects. Updating the Widmark Equation. *J Stud Alcohol* 1981;42:547-56.

Wedel M, Pieters JE, Pikaar NA et al. Application of a three-compartment model to a study of the effects of sex, alcohol dose and concentration, exercise and food consumption on the pharmacokinetics of ethanol in healthy volunteers. *Alcohol Alcohol* 1991;26:329-36.

West, R. *Theory of addiction.* Oxford, UK: Blackwell Publishing, 2006.

White HR, Marmorstein NR, Crews FT et al. Associations between heavy drinking and changes in impulsive behavior among adolescent boys. *Alcohol Clin Exp Res* 2011;35:295-303.

Williams EC, Rubinsky AD, Chavez LJ et al. An early evaluation of implementation of brief intervention for unhealthy alcohol use in the US Veterans Health Administration. *Addiction* 2014;109(9):1472-81.

Winograd RP, Littlefield AK, Martinez J et al. The drunken self: the five-factor model as an organizational framework for characterizing perceptions of one's own drunkenness. *Alcohol Clin Exp Res* 2012;36:1787-93.

Yeomans H. Blurred visions: experts, evidence and the promotion of moderate drinking. *Sociological Rev* 2013;24:62:S2:58 - 78.

Index

AA...143, 149, 153, 161
Abbreviations..10
Abstinence, lifelong...47
Acetaldehyde...118p.
Acetaldehyde dehydrogenase (ALDH)......................................55
Addiction...141
Aggression.....................................93, 113, 125, 141, 197
Alcohol addiction...141
Alcohol dehydrogenase (AHD)...54
Alcohol dependence...141
Alcohol intake..23
Alcohol-specific disease..175
Alcoholics Anonymous (AA)..143
Ambivalence...159
American Cancer Society Study.......................................34, 119
Anti-alcohol academics...45
AUDIT...98, 100pp.
Availability..188
Baboons...115
BAC...61pp., 66
Bailey Scales of Infant Development.......................................133
Beer..........15, 23, 63, 73, 76, 79pp., 88p., 91, 98, 108, 122, 195

Blood pressure............................20, 42, 57p., 83pp., 122
Body weight................................42, 62p., 66, 77, 116
Breast cancer...50, 120
Breath-analyzers...129
Brief advice.....................................98, 100, 104pp.
Britain..106, 134
Cancer...118
Changes in alcohol intake.....................................50
Churchill, Winston.......................................14, 58
CI...22, 34, 80, 120, 188
Coffee..15, 76, 83pp., 117, 141
Confidence interval..10, 22
Confounding..19
Constructivism...47
Craving.....................................141, 143p., 149, 165
Diagnostic and Statistical Manual of Mental Disorders..........10
Diagnostic criteria......................................132, 143
Dietary energy..20
Discounting...157p.
Disease concept..143
Drapetomania..146
Drink...23
Drinking rhythm...27, 81
DSM.......................104, 143, 145p., 167, 188
Elizabeth II...39
Energy value..42, 72
Epictetus..153, 165

Essentialistic trap...177
FAS...132
Fetal alcohol spectrum disorder...131
Fetal alcohol syndrome...131
Fibrinogen..50, 58
Finland...48, 57, 175pp., 179
Flavor..87, 91p.
France...37, 70, 131, 175, 185, 195
Francis of Assisi...153
Free will..157
Gamma-glutamyltransferase (GGT)..98
Genes...88, 120, 136, 149pp.
Gout..122
Grand Rapids Study..129
Habit loop..146, 164p.
HDL...52p.
Heart disease...............20, 26p., 43, 52, 58, 81, 84p., 122, 164
Hepatitis...116
Heuristics...21, 158
High-density lipoprotein..10
Homosexuality..146
ICD..145, 175p.
Incidence...18
International Classification of Diseases...................................10
Intoxication...........26p., 60, 70p., 93, 135, 156, 167p., 180, 217
Ireland...176p.
Irregular pattern..30

J-shape..25, 48

LDL..52, 84

Life-span..16, 57

Lifelong abstainers..47

Lincoln, Abraham...181

Liquor............................5, 15, 23, 63, 76, 80pp., 108, 140, 195

Liver cirrhosis...114, 176

Liver enzymes..99

Lognormal model..185

Loss of control......................................143p., 149, 152

Mendelian randomization..54

Meta-analysis.................22, 26, 34, 52p., 58, 119, 132p., 170

Million Women Study..120

Moral panic...136

Mortality of alcoholics...170, 187

Natural experiments..194

North Korea...196

Oriental people.......................................55, 119, 150

Pearl, Raymond...19

PH...78p., 123

Placebo...70, 170

Plato...40

Poisoning..60, 69, 77, 194

Price..188

Professional treatment..169

Prohibition..19, 140p., 145, 174, 195

Randomized..51p., 70, 84, 105

Randomized controlled trial...51p.

Rat...57, 94, 115, 151p.

Record your alcohol intake...................................107

Recovery...167

Relative risk..........................11, 22, 27p., 34, 42p., 130, 175

Reward.......................................153, 157, 159, 165pp.

Risk..21, 42

Risk level..33

Risky drinking...24

RR..43

Safe level..33

Scientific Perspectivism..46

Self-help.................................124, 142, 166p., 171

Self-rated health...28

Serenity Prayer...153

Skewed distribution..184

Smoking......20, 27, 43, 88, 100, 116pp., 135, 141, 163p., 187p.

Social construction..146p.

Steady intake..30

Supertaster...88

Taste..........................75p., 78p., 82, 84, 86pp., 93, 157

Tea..15, 76, 80, 83pp.

Temptation...159pp., 165

Time-series..185

Tolerance..68p., 128, 143

Total consumption model.............................181, 196

Traffic accidents...128

Uncertainty..22, 58
Underestimation...37
Underreporting..37
Underreporting, alcohol.......................................37
USA....19, 47, 61, 70, 105, 108, 120, 136, 141, 143, 146p., 188, 190p., 195p.
Utilities..112, 157
Warning labels..136
Water......................5, 15, 61pp., 72, 76pp., 82, 84p., 93, 122p.
Wine..........15, 23, 63p., 71, 76, 79pp., 86pp., 95, 108, 122, 195
Witchcraft..146

Printed in Great Britain
by Amazon